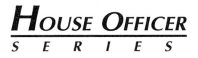

HOUSE OFFICER
S E R I E S

Neurology

SEVENTH EDITION

W9-AOW-335

Dedication

To our wives, Mira, Eva, and Mary Bruce

HOUSE OFFICER
S E R I E S

Neurology

SEVENTH EDITION

Howard L. Weiner, M.D.

Department of Neurology
Center for Neurologic Diseases
Brigham & Women's Hospital
Harvard Medical School
Boston, Massachusetts

Lawrence P. Levitt, M.D.

Division of Neurology
Lehigh Valley Hospital
Allentown, Pennsylvania

Alexander D. Rae-Grant, M.D.

Division of Neurology
Lehigh Valley Hospital
Allentown, Pennsylvania

The House Officer Series is based on Weiner and Levitt's *Neurology for the House Officer*, first published in 1973.

 LIPPINCOTT WILLIAMS & WILKINS
A **Wolters Kluwer** Company
Philadelphia · Baltimore · New York · London
Buenos Aires · Hong Kong · Sydney · Tokyo

Acquisitions Editor: Charles W. Mitchell
Developmental Editor: Scott Scheidt
Production Editor: Emily Lerman
Manufacturing Manager: Colin J. Warnock
Cover Designer: David Levy
Compositor: Lippincott Williams & Wilkins Desktop Division
Printer: R. R. Donnelley–Crawfordsville

Library of Congress Cataloging-in-Publication Data

Weiner, Howard L.
    Neurology / Howard L. Weiner, Lawrence P. Levitt, Alexander D. Rae-Grant.—7th ed.
      p. ; cm.—(House officer series)
    Includes bibliographical references and index.
    ISBN 0-7817-4747-3 (alk. paper)
    1. Nervous system—Diseases—Handbooks, manuals, etc. 2. Neurology—
Handbooks, manuals, etc. I. Levitt, Lawrence P., 1940– II. Rae-Grant, Alexander D.
III. Title. IV. Series.
    [DNLM: 1. Nervous System Diseases. 2. Neurologic Manifestations.
WL 140 W423n 2004]
RC355.W44 2004
616.8—dc22

                                                                    2003065870

Care has been taken to confirm the accuracy of the information presented and to describe generally accepted practices. However, the authors and publisher are not responsible for errors or
omissions or for any consequences from application of the information in this book and make
no warranty, expressed or implied, with respect to the currency, completeness, or accuracy of
the contents of the publication. Application of this information in a particular situation remains
the professional responsibility of the practitioner.

The authors and publisher have exerted every effort to ensure that drug selection and dosage
set forth in this text are in accordance with current recommendations and practice at the time of
publication. However, in view of ongoing research, changes in government regulations, and the
constant flow of information relating to drug therapy and drug reactions, the reader is urged to
check the package insert for each drug for any change in indications and dosage and for added
warnings and precautions. This is particularly important when the recommended agent is a new
or infrequently employed drug.

Some drugs and medical devices presented in this publication have Food and Drug Administration (FDA) clearance for limited use in restricted research settings. It is the responsibility of
the health care provider to ascertain the FDA status of each drug or device planned for use in
their clinical practice.

10 9 8 7 6 5 4 3 2 1

Foreword

It is a daunting task to write a foreword to a classic. Ever since I can remember, house staff and students on a neurology service were carrying in their white coat pockets *Neurology for the House Officer* by Howard L. Weiner and Lawrence P. Levitt. The first edition, published over 30 years ago, immediately filled an enormous need. Bright house officers nimble in general medicine, cardiology, infectious diseases, nephrology, and the like, were surprisingly weak in neurology. Although patients with neurologic problems were common on the wards and in the clinics of general hospitals, young physicians were poorly prepared to evaluate and treat such people. Everyone seemed to need the clearly written, straightforward, and practical approach of Drs. Levitt and Weiner, which had grown out of practical experience at the then Peter Bent Brigham Hospital.

An entire generation of physicians has learned basic neurology from this remarkable little book. It is fair to say that no other single work has had such an enormous impact on the neurologic education of doctors who are now practicing, mostly as non-neurologists, with an incrementally better understanding of the basic principles of neurology evaluation based on history taking and localization. The book has spawned an entire genre of house officer manuals and has been widely imitated, but never surpassed.

Now the authors have included case material to support the text and have incorporated new technology and the latest therapy into their discussion of neurologic diagnosis and therapy. The important thing is that the skeleton remains: a careful history to determine the pace of the illness and a focused neurologic examination aimed at determining the location of the lesion. After 30 years of incredible change in virtually every aspect of medical care, it is reassuring to note the white coats of house officers and students rotating on the neurology service still contain the familiar little bible, *Neurology for the House Officer.*

Martin A. Samuels, M.D., F.A.C.P., F.A.A.N.

Martin A. Samuels, M.D., F.A.C.P., F.A.A.N., is Professor of Neurology at the Harvard Medical School and Chair of the Department of Neurology at the Brigham and Women's Hospital. He received his B.A. from Williams College in 1967 and his M.D. from the University of Cincinnati College of Medicine in 1971. Dr. Samuels completed an internship, residency, and chief residency in Internal Medicine at Boston City Hospital and Neurology Residency at the Massachusetts General Hospital. He was Chief of the Neurology Service at the Brockton–West Roxbury VA Medical Center for 11 years before assuming the position as Chief of Neurology at the Brigham and Women's Hospital and Director of the Harvard–Longwood Neurology Training Program in 1988. In 1996, Dr. Samuels became the founding Chair of the Department of Neurology at the Brigham and Women's Hospital and Co-director of Partners Neurology. He is the editor of the *Manual of Neurologic Therapeutics,* seven editions, the neurology section of *Stein's Internal Medicine,* 3rd and 4th editions, *Office Practice of Neurology,* two editions, *Hospitalist Neurology,* and author of the *Video Textbook of Neurology for the Practicing Physician.* He has won numerous prizes for teaching, including the first Harvard Medical School Faculty Prize for Excellence in Teaching. Dr. Samuels is board certified in Internal Medicine and Neurology, and his special interest is the interface between these specialties.

Foreword to the First Edition (1973)

Having spent my professional life in a teaching hospital with a steady stream of students, house officers, and residents, I have gradually become accustomed to the varying neurologic backgrounds of these young physicians.

The neurologist and the internist exhibit significant differences in approach. The internist is usually trained to think physiologically in terms of the meaning and cause of specific symptoms. The neurologist, on the other hand, brings to the patient encounter not only his history and physical examination, but also a special "neurologic examination." This special examination is designed more to answer the question "where is the lesion" than "what is wrong with the patient." The neurologist, therefore, can profit tremendously from a knowledge of neuroanatomy and neurophysiology combined with a careful neurologic examination and appropriate evaluation.

In this country, most students and medical residents, general practitioners, and internists do not develop strong backgrounds in neurology. They therefore profit less from their neurologic endeavors than they might. Nevertheless, they are still required to care for patients with nervous system disorders and are often significantly insecure about treatment.

In attempting to deal with this problem, two of our most capable neurology residents, Howard L. Weiner, M.D., and Lawrence P. Levitt, M.D., began compiling notes from their lectures to small groups of students. This soon became source material for future reference. The demand for this material grew geometrically and was widely used by students and residents. The need for a practical manual was appreciated, and the authors began a more systematic approach to problems with which they were recurrently faced on the wards of a large teaching hospital. As fast as they could put the sections out, students, medical interns, and residents kept requesting them, and soon large numbers were being duplicated. The material was recognized for its practical and common sense approach to problems frequently encountered.

After 2 years of intense effort to gather constructive suggestions, find unmet needs, and weed out unimportant material, the authors have written this handbook.

It was originally planned for local use in our hospitals and given to students and residents rotating through the service. As requests for the handbook began to arrive from many areas, the need for wider circulation was appreciated. This need was translated into the decision to publish this handbook.

Since it has been so enthusiastically received by critical students and residents here, we believe it will meet the practical needs of young physicians elsewhere.

H. Richard Tyler, M.D.

About the Authors

Howard L. Weiner, M.D., is Physician in Medicine (Neurology) at the Brigham and Women's Hospital and Robert L. Kroc Professor of Neurology at Harvard Medical School. He attended Dartmouth College and the University of Colorado Medical School. He then interned at Chaim Sheba Hospital, Tel Hashomer, Israel, and served as a medical resident at the Beth Israel Hospital, Boston. He received his neurology training at the Harvard teaching hospitals of the Longwood Area Neurology Program. Dr. Weiner is Director of the Partners Multiple Sclerosis program at the Brigham and Women's and Massachusetts General Hospitals and Co-Director of the Center for Neurologic Diseases at the Brigham and Women's Hospital.

Lawrence P. Levitt, M.D., is Senior Consultant Emeritus in Neurology at Lehigh Valley Hospital in Allentown, Pennsylvania. He is a Professor of Clinical Neurology at Penn State College of Medicine. A graduate of Queens College, he then attended Cornell Medical College as a Jonas Salk Scholar. Dr. Levitt interned and was a first-year medical resident at Bellevue Hospital; he then spent 2 years in the Public Health Service at the Encephalitis Research Center in Tampa, Florida. He did his neurology training at the Harvard teaching hospitals of the Longwood Area Neurology Program.

Alexander D. Rae-Grant, M.D., is the President of the medical staff, Lehigh Valley Hospital, Allentown, Pennsylvania. He is an Associate Professor of Clinical Medicine at Penn State College of Medicine. A graduate of Yale University, he attended McMaster University Medical School in Ontario. He was a medical resident at Sunnybrook Hospital of the University of Toronto, and did his neurology training at the University of Western Ontario in London, Ontario.

Preface

Neurology for the House Officer is designed to help physicians properly recognize and treat neurologic diseases. It is not meant to be a complete survey, but is an attempt to provide a succinct and lucid approach to common neurologic problems. The seventh edition has been rewritten to incorporate the many changes in neurologic practice over the past 5 years. In the suggested readings, we have identified pivotal trials, well-written reviews, and important clinical observations to provide the reader easy access to more detailed descriptions of neurologic illness.

Our approach continues to be problem-oriented: how to deal with a patient who is comatose, who has a right hemiplegia, or who is demented. We continue to try to make neurologic diagnosis and treatment an accessible, understandable subject for students and residents as well as non-neurologists. We are gratified by the widespread use of previous editions and hope that the seventh edition continues to fill the need for a readable, "carry-in-the-pocket" practical reference to neurologic illness.

Howard L. Weiner, M.D.
Lawrence P. Levitt, M.D.
Alexander D. Rae-Grant, M.D.

Acknowledgments

This manual was reviewed by students and house officers at the Harvard teaching hospitals of the Partners Neurology Program (Brigham and Women's Hospital and the Massachusetts General Hospital). It was also reviewed by neurology residents at the University of Western Ontario. We are grateful to them for their encouragement, enthusiasm, and advice, and for identifying those neurologic problems and concepts most important to them. We thank the following for their help in reviewing the manuscript: Yvette Bordelon, Bradford Dickerson, Leigh Hochberg, and Christen Shoesmith. In addition, individual chapters were reviewed by John Castaldo, Marc Dichter, Timothy Friel, and Dennis Selkoe, and we are grateful for their expert assistance.

Contents

   The neurologic examination is designed to establish the
   localization of dysfunction in the nervous system. Many
   processes affect only specific areas in the nervous system.
   Thus, anatomic localization becomes the foundation for
   diagnosis and treatment.

   Right-sided weakness may be secondary to a lesion affecting
   the pyramidal tract anywhere from cortex to spinal cord.
   Evaluation of associated signs and symptoms—e.g., aphasia
   with cortical lesions—is made to determine the level of the
   lesion.

   Denial of illness and inattention of the left side are major
   features of nondominant hemisphere dysfunction. Tests of
   spatial organization and attention replace aphasia testing in
   evaluating patients with left hemiplegia.

   Aphasia is the major feature of dominant hemisphere dysfunction. Recognition of aphasia establishes the level of nervous system involvement, and characterization may suggest
   the etiology.

The clinical diagnosis of coma requires delineation of the
nature and degree of central nervous system dysfunction.
This chapter presents an approach to examining and evaluating the comatose patient.

In the patient with dizziness, the physician must establish
whether the problem is peripheral (labyrinth), central (e.g.,
brainstem), or systemic (e.g., cardiac). Newer treatments for
positional vertigo are discussed.

Evaluation of the deep tendon reflexes provides a valuable
screen of the nervous system. This chapter outlines those disease processes producing hyperreflexia (pyramidal tract dysfunction).

Decreased reflexes imply disease affecting the reflex arc. Disorders that diminish reflexes, particularly peripheral neuropathies, are discussed.

Acute spinal cord compression is a neurologic emergency.
There are characteristic symptoms and signs. Treatment
must be rapid and diagnosis of the cause is crucial.

Neuroanatomy forms the foundation for evaluating the
patient with nerve and root dysfunction. An abbreviated
course of the most commonly used anatomic facts is presented, with a discussion of the most common nerve and
root injuries and their clinical significance.

The physician must establish whether weakness is indeed
myopathic—whether the myopathy is congenital or
acquired—and if acquired, whether it represents a manifestation of another illness (e.g., thyroid myopathy).

Chapter 1

Localization

One of the major features of neurologic diagnosis is *localization of the lesion* in the nervous system. This approach is needed if one is to arrive consistently at reasonable diagnoses. Anatomic orientation is not merely an intellectual exercise; knowing where the lesion is often will indicate what it is, will help guide in management, and will be crucial in deciding on diagnostic procedures. These examples illustrate the utility of localization in diagnosis.

PURE MOTOR HEMIPLEGIA

The nature of its anatomy usually defines the vascular lesion as a lacune and means that arteriography, anticoagulation, and surgery usually are not indicated. For more information regarding pure motor hemiplegia, see Chapter 16.

MULTIPLE SCLEROSIS

Multiple lesions in the nervous system and a history of exacerbations and remissions are required for the diagnosis. When patients are misdiagnosed as having multiple sclerosis, there is often only one anatomic lesion.

HYSTERICAL SYMPTOMS

A conversion disorder (hysteria) is suspected when symptoms and/or signs do not fit anatomic rules.

FOOT-DROP

Foot-drop can be seen with peripheral nerve, nerve root, spinal cord, or hemisphere disease. One must decide where the dysfunction is before beginning investigation.

IS THE NERVOUS SYSTEM INVOLVED?

Although this may appear self-evident, some of the most difficult problems in neurologic diagnosis can occur when the answer to a "neurologic problem" lies *outside* the nervous system. Examples include a patient who has nonepileptic seizures (pseudoseizures) and who is treated with intubation and intravenous lorazepam, a patient treated for sciatica who has an occult femoral neck fracture, or a patient with "acute cervical radiculopathy" who actually has "atypical angina."

Knowledge of detailed neuroanatomy is usually unnecessary to decide whether the lesion is cortical or subcortical or in the brainstem, spinal cord, peripheral nerve, or muscle. When necessary, anatomic localization can be refined—first with the help of this manual and later with textbooks. The major obstacle in making neurologic diagnoses will have been overcome if, after completing the history and physical examination, the physician begins the analysis by asking "Where is the lesion?"

Suggested Reading

Brazis PW, Masdeu JC, Biller J. *Localization in clinical neurology*, 3rd ed. Boston: Little, Brown and Company, 1996.

Gilman S, Winans-Newman S. *Manter and Gantz's essentials of clinical neuroanatomy and neurophysiology*, 7th ed. Philadelphia: FA Davis, 1987.

Chapter 2

Right Hemiplegia

When examining a patient who has right hemiplegia (paralysis) or right hemiparesis (weakness), establish whether the lesion is cortical, subcortical, in the brainstem, or in the spinal cord (Fig. 2.1).

IS THE LESION CORTICAL?

1. Test the patient carefully for *aphasia* (a disorder of production or comprehension of language). Listen to spontaneous speech. Note any breakdown in fluency. Notice any errors of word or syllable choice (paraphasias). Have the patient name objects (e.g., pen, tie, watch), repeat phrases ("no ifs, ands, or buts"), and read. Check the patient's comprehension of commands ("Touch your left thumb to your right ear. Close your eyes."). Have the patient write a sentence or two. Is the patient right handed? Remember, in nearly all right-handed and most left-handed people, the left hemisphere is dominant for language (see Chapter 4).
2. Check for *cortical sensory loss.* Test position sense, graphesthesia (write numbers on the palm), and stereognosis (have the patient identify objects placed in the hand). Touch the patient on different parts of the arm and leg and have him or her identify where he or she was touched. Touch both sides at the same time to see if the patient notices one side only (extinction). Remember, primary sensation (pin, touch, temperature) must be intact to do such testing. Cortical sen-

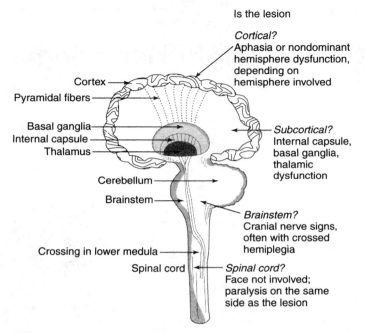

Is the lesion

Cortical?
Aphasia or nondominant
hemisphere dysfunction,
depending on
hemisphere involved

Cortex

Pyramidal fibers

Basal ganglia
Internal capsule
Thalamus

Subcortical?
Internal capsule,
basal ganglia,
thalamic
dysfunction

Cerebellum

Brainstem

Brainstem?
Cranial nerve signs,
often with crossed
hemiplegia

Crossing in lower medulla

Spinal cord

Spinal cord?
Face not involved;
paralysis on the same
side as the lesion

FIGURE 2.1. Establishing the level of the lesion in a patient with hemiplegia. Upper motor neurons located in the frontal and parietal cortex course
down through the subcortical white matter, into the internal capsule, and
through the brainstem and then cross in the lower medulla to the opposite
side (decussation of the pyramids). They descend in the lateral spinal cord to
synapse in the anterior horn with the lower motor neuron.

sory loss implies a parietal or subcortical localization on the
contralateral side.
3. Are the *face and arm are more affected than the leg* (suggesting
   middle cerebral artery territory in a stroke patient) or is the
   leg is more involved (frontal lobe or anterior cerebral artery
   territory)?
4. Is there *eye deviation* or a gaze preference? Do the eyes look
   toward the hemisphere involved and away from the hemiparesis in a cortical lesion (see Fig. 34.3)?
5. Check carefully for a *field defect*. Ask the patient to identify
   fingers presented simultaneously in peripheral fields. *Note:*

Field defects and "cortical-type" eye deviation may be found in subcortical lesions and must be interpreted in the context of other findings. The presence of seizures, cortical sensory loss, or aphasia often will assist in accurate diagnosis.

6. *Are there seizures?* A hemiparesis associated with a seizure suggests a cortical lesion. Has the patient had seizures in the same distribution as the weakness?

IS THE LESION SUBCORTICAL?

Subcortical structures include the internal capsule, basal ganglia (globus pallidus and putamen), and thalamus.

1. Are the *face, arm, and leg equally involved* (characteristic of lesions in the internal capsule)? Is there sparing of speech despite a hemiparesis, suggesting sparing of left hemisphere cortex?

2. Are there unusual movements or *dystonic postures* (seen with basal ganglia lesions)?

3. Is there a *dense sensory loss* to pin and touch in the face, arm, and leg (seen with thalamic lesions) associated with the hemiplegia (involvement of the adjacent internal capsule)? *Note:* The sensory loss often splits the midline.

4. Is there visual field defect (seen with lesions of the optic tracts or optic radiations)?

IS THE LESION IN THE BRAINSTEM?

1. Look for *crossed hemiplegia*, a classic feature of brainstem lesions. Right hemiplegia from a left-sided brainstem lesion often is accompanied by left-sided brainstem signs (e.g., left-sided dysmetria or cranial nerve palsies) at the level of the lesion.

2. Check for *ataxia*: finger-to-nose ataxia, difficulty with rapid alternating movements in the limbs, or difficulty walking heel-to-toe (tandem gait). Such ataxia may suggest a cerebellar or brainstem lesion. Remember, limb ataxia is almost always on the same side as the lesion, so a left brainstem lesion gives left limb ataxia. Do not misinterpret weakness for ataxia.

3. Note *nystagmus.* Horizontal nystagmus is usually more marked when the patient gazes toward the side of the lesion.

Vertical nystagmus is more specific for brainstem and cerebellar disease than is horizontal nystagmus.

4. Check for *hearing loss*, which occurs in the ear opposite the hemiparesis. Ask about *vertigo*, which suggests a lesion in the brainstem or cerebellum.

5. Check carefully for *sensory findings*. Characteristic findings are pain, temperature, and corneal loss on the left side of the face (involvement of descending tract of the fifth nerve) with pain and temperature loss on the right side of the body (spinothalamic tract).

6. Note *dysarthria* (slurred speech) and *dysphagia* (difficulty swallowing), which may be caused by disorders of the ninth and tenth cranial nerves (lower motor neuron) or the corticobulbar fibers supplying them (upper motor neuron). A decreased gag reflex is seen with lower motor neuron lesions. Upper motor neuron involvement causes a pseudobulbar palsy (hyperactive gag, brisk jaw jerk, and emotional lability).

7. Check for abnormal *eye movements*. In left brainstem lesions, the patient may have trouble looking to the left (gaze paresis) (see Fig. 34.4), may have eye deviation to the right, or may have problems adducting the left eye (internuclear ophthalmoplegia) (see Fig. 34.8).

8. In *twelfth nerve lesions*, the tongue deviates to the side of the lesion. Thus, in a left twelfth nerve lesion, the tongue deviates to the left as the stronger muscles on the right force the tongue left. Use the tip of the nose as a reference point. See how fast the tongue can move back and forth. Upper motor lesions slow tongue movements, leaving tongue bulk normal, whereas lower motor neuron lesions cause tongue atrophy on the affected side.

IS THE LESION IN THE SPINAL CORD?

1. The *face* is spared except for high cervical cord lesions, in which there is facial pain and temperature loss as a result of involvement of the trigeminal nerve, which descends one or two segments into the cervical cord.

2. Weakness is usually bilateral. If unilateral, vibration and position loss are on the same side as weakness, but pain and tem-

perature are affected on the opposite side (Brown-Séquard syndrome) (see Fig. 34.10).
3. A *sensory level* to pin, vibration, or sweating may be found and is most characteristic of a spinal cord lesion.
4. *Bladder and bowel* disturbances are common.
5. *Cranial nerves are spared.* Rarely, the spinal tract of the trigeminal nerve may be affected in high spinal cord lesions. The sympathetic supply to the pupil descends through the cord to T1 or T2, so a Horner's syndrome may occur in cervical cord lesions and high thoracic cord lesions.

Suggested Reading

Brazis PW, Masdeu JC, Biller J. *Localization in clinical neurology,* 3rd ed. Boston: Little, Brown and Company, 1996.

Gilman S, Winans-Newman S. *Manter and Gatz's essentials of clinical neuroanatomy and neurophysiology,* 7th ed. Philadelphia: FA Davis, 1987.

Chapter 3

Left Hemiplegia

When examining a patient with a left hemiplegia or hemiparesis, nondominant hemisphere function rather than aphasia testing is stressed. The remainder of cortical, subcortical, brainstem, and spinal cord testing is the same as the testing involved with right hemiplegia.

ARE THERE NONDOMINANT HEMISPHERE FINDINGS?

1. Check for inattention. Does the patient neglect the body's left side, the left side of the room, or the left side of a picture? Check for extinction by double simultaneous tactile or visual stimulation (touch both of the patient's hands at once and ask which was touched; have the patient identify fingers presented simultaneously in left and right visual fields).

2. Check for denial or "lack of concern." Does the patient say there is nothing wrong, despite having a hemiplegia, or does the patient show a lack of concern? Sometimes, a patient will identify the patient's left hand as belonging to someone else or as the examiner's hand when it is lifted into view. These are elements of anosognosia (the denial of a neurologic deficit).

3. Test for constructional apraxia. Have the patient copy a simple diagram such as a bicycle, car, or house. Have the patient draw a clock and fill in the numbers. Drawing complex figures will bring out parietal deficits missed by many other tests.

4. Check for spatial disorientation. Does the patient get lost in the hospital or when driving in his or her neighborhood? Lead the patient from the room. Can he or she find the way back? Can the patient figure out directions for local travel?

5. Is the patient acutely confused (reported with some nondominant hemisphere strokes)?

6. Is there a loss of the melody and emotional content of speech or thought? Nondominant lesions may rob patients of the ability to express or understand emotional speech and make them unresponsive to usual emotional stimuli (aprosody).

7. Does the patient give up on tasks? Motor impersistence may be seen in nondominant frontal lesions. Can the tongue be held out or an "ahhh" maintained?

8. Does the patient have difficulty dressing? Nondominant parietal lesions may cause a dressing apraxia.

Suggested Reading

Critchley M. The parietal lobes. In: Denny-Brown D, Chambers RA, eds. *The parietal lobe and behavior.* New York: Hafner, 1969.

Fisher CM. Left hemiplegia and motor impersistence. *J Nerv Ment Dis* 1956;123:201.

Mesulam M-M, Waxman S, Geschwind N, et al. Acute confusional states with right middle cerebral artery infarctions. *J Neurol Neurosurg Psychiatry* 1976;39:84.

Chapter 4

Aphasia

Aphasia is a disorder of language. The patient with aphasia uses language incorrectly or comprehends it imperfectly. In contrast, the patient with dysarthria articulates poorly, but grammar and word choice are correct. Aphasia may show up as difficulty finding words, using the wrong words, having trouble repeating, or having trouble understanding what others say. Aphasia must be recognized clinically because it localizes the lesion to the cortex (or immediately under the cortex) and usually to the left hemisphere. There are three exceptions:

1. Some (fewer than 50%) left-handed people use the right hemisphere for speech.
2. Anomic aphasias, in which the inability to generate word names is the predominant feature, may result from metabolic disorders or space-occupying lesions with pressure effects.
3. Basal ganglia and thalamic lesions, especially in the left hemisphere, may produce aphasia.

Because different types of aphasia may imply different localizations, the clinician first must recognize that aphasia exists and then characterize it.

ANATOMY OF APHASIA

Language "ability" is a function of the left hemisphere for almost all right-handed and for most left-handed individuals. The "language areas" are located in the distribution of the middle cere-

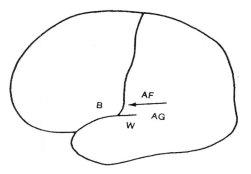

FIGURE 4.1.   The primary regions of speech production. Moving from posterior to anterior, they are Wernicke's area (*W*) or the posterior part of the first temporal gyrus, the angular gyrus (*AG*), the arcuate fasciculus (*AF*), and Broca's area (*B*) or the posterior third frontal gyrus.

bral artery surrounding the Sylvian fissure (frontal and temporal cortex). Important areas for speech include Broca's area of the inferior frontal lobe, Wernicke's area in the superior temporal lobe, the arcuate fasciculus, the supramarginal gyrus, and the nearby cortex (Fig. 4.1).

Broca's and Wernicke's areas are connected by the arcuate fasciculus. *Wernicke's area* lies next to the primary auditory cortex and involves the "understanding" of auditory input as language and monitors speech output. It is connected with the *supramarginal gyrus*, a center for integrating sensory and other association information.

The arcuate fasciculus is a white-matter tract leading to *Broca's area*, which, in turn, is responsible for the motor part or "production" of language. Broca's area helps translate the information carried from other language areas into phonation and speech output.

TYPES OF APHASIA

Although there is a continuum of aphasia and its severity, patients with aphasia can be subcategorized, depending on the type of problem they have. These subcategories have anatomic and pathologic significance.

Broca's Aphasia

With Broca's aphasia, the lesion is in or near Broca's area (inferior frontal cortex near the motor strip).

1. Speech is *nonfluent* (halting), produced with great effort, and poorly articulated. There is marked reduction in total speech, which may be "telegraphic" with the omission of articles (the, an) or word endings.
2. *Comprehension* of written and verbal speech is good, except where grammar is required. For example, a patient may have difficulty with a question such as "if a tiger is eaten by a lion, which one is still alive?"
3. *Repetition* of single words may be good, although it is done with great effort; phrase repetition is poor, especially phrases containing words such as "if, " "and, " or "but. "
4. The patient always *writes* in an aphasic manner, and writing is affected even in a subtle aphasia.
5. *Object naming* is usually poor, although it may be better than spontaneous speech.
6. *Hemiparesis* (usually greater in the face and arm than the leg) is present in larger lesions because the motor cortex is close to Broca's area.
7. The patient is *aware* of this deficit, but is frustrated and frequently depressed.
8. Interestingly, the patient may be able to *hum a melody* normally. However, a musician may have deficits in producing music. Curses or other ejaculatory speech may be well articulated. These exceptions are the result of right-hemisphere mechanisms for such emotional speech.
9. Buccolingual apraxia, which is difficulty producing facial movements to command not caused by poor comprehension or paralysis, may be present. It is demonstrated by having the patient try to protrude the tongue, blow out the cheeks, or whistle.

Wernicke's Aphasia

With Wernicke's aphasia, the lesion is in or near Wernicke's area of the dominant temporal lobe.

1. *Speech is fluent* with normal rhythm and articulation, but it conveys information poorly because of meandering, indirect

phrases (circumlocutions) and use of nonsense words (neologisms) and incorrect words (paraphasic errors).

2. The patient uses wrong words and sounds. For example: "letter" for "ladder" (phonemic paraphasia) or "orange" for "apple" (semantic paraphasia).
3. The patient is unable to *comprehend* written or verbal speech.
4. The content of *writing* is abnormal, as is speech, although the penmanship may be good.
5. *Repetition* is poor.
6. *Object naming* is poor.
7. *Hemiparesis* is mild or absent because the lesion is far from the motor cortex. A hemianopsia or quadrantanopsia may be present owing to involvement of optic radiations passing through the affected temporal lobe.
8. Patients do not realize the nature of their deficit and usually are not depressed in the acute stage. They may exhibit elements of paranoia for this reason.
9. This type of aphasia is commonly the result of an embolic event to the superior temporal gyrus.

Conduction Aphasia

Conduction aphasia is caused by a lesion in the posterior part of the superior temporal gyrus or supramarginal gyrus and functionally disconnects the anterior and posterior speech areas.

1. *Speech* is fluent but conveys information imperfectly. Paraphasic errors are common.
2. The patient can *comprehend* spoken or written phrases containing small grammatical words.
3. *Repetition* is the most severely affected, especially for phrases containing grammatical words and nonsense syllables.
4. There is difficulty *naming objects.*
5. *Written language* is impaired, although penmanship is preserved.
6. *Hemiparesis*, if present, is mild.

Anomic Aphasia

1. Anomic aphasia may be seen with small lesions in the angular gyrus, toxic or metabolic encephalopathies, or focal space-occupying lesions far from the speech area that exert

pressure effects. It is the least localizing of the aphasias and should prompt a serious search for reversible, metabolic causes. It is a common manifestation of Alzheimer's disease.

2. *Speech* is fluent but conveys information poorly because of paraphasic errors and circumlocutions. (Literally, patients talk around words they cannot recall.) The main problem is naming. This can be demonstrated by having the patient name as many animals as possible in 1 minute. A person should be able to name 10 or more.

3. The patient can *understand* written and spoken speech.

4. There is no *hemiplegia.*

5. *Comprehension* and *repetition* are normal, although these may be difficult to assess in a patient who is confused (e.g., in metabolic encephalopathy).

Global Aphasia

Global aphasia is seen with large lesions affecting both Wernicke's and Broca's areas. Marked hemiparesis occurs, in addition to inability to comprehend and to speak. Global aphasia is seen with large infarcts in the middle cerebral artery territory and often is caused by occlusion of the left internal carotid artery or trunk of the middle cerebral artery.

Other Aphasic Syndromes

Aphasias may occur because of lesions located outside the perisylvian region, in "border zone" areas. These "transcortical aphasias" are characterized by a relative sparing of repetition despite other language difficulties. The clinical importance of transcortical aphasias is that they typically are related to prolonged hypotension or hypoxia (e.g., after cardiac arrest). These patients often repeat and read well, but have diminished fluency (anterior border zone lesions) or comprehend poorly (posterior border zone lesions).

EXAMINATION OF THE PATIENT WITH APHASIA

First establish whether the patient is aphasic, then determine the nature of the aphasia. Remember, it may be difficult to determine whether a patient who is inattentive or confused is aphasic.

1. *Listen to speech output.* Is it fluent or nonfluent? If fluent, the lesion is posterior; if nonfluent, it usually is anterior.

2. Can the patient *read and write* without errors? If so, aphasia is not present.
3. Check *naming*. In the patient with aphasia, naming almost always is impaired.
4. Check for *repetition*. If the patient is aphasic but can repeat, there is a transcortical aphasia.
5. Can the patient comprehend simple yes or no questions? Comprehension is relatively spared in Broca's aphasia.
6. Is there *hemiparesis*? If so, the lesion is anterior, involving the motor area.
7. To delineate the various types of fluent aphasias, check whether the patient can repeat and comprehend.
   - Wernicke's: cannot repeat or comprehend
   - Conduction: cannot repeat, but can comprehend
   - Anomic: can repeat and comprehend

THE IMPORTANCE OF DEFINING THE APHASIA

The definition of aphasia localizes the *level* of the nervous system lesion. If aphasia is present, the lesion is usually in the left cerebral cortex. Someone with difficulty using the right hand and a mild aphasia has hemisphere disease, not a brachial plexus lesion.

Aphasia on a vascular basis implies dysfunction of middle cerebral artery territory and often is caused by disease of the internal carotid in the neck. Marked stenosis of the internal carotid may be surgically correctable, and if recognized and treated in time, a mild or transient aphasia may be prevented from becoming global.

The sudden onset of fluent aphasia without hemiparesis often means an embolus to the posterior branch of the middle cerebral artery. Look for an embolic focus in the heart or in the carotid artery. If the heart is the source, anticoagulation should be considered; if the carotid is the suspected source, angiography usually is performed in search of a surgically remediable lesion. Remember the clinical rule: the sudden onset of aphasia without hemiparesis suggests embolus.

PROGNOSIS

The prognosis of aphasia in a given patient depends on the location and extent of the lesion, as well as the underlying pathology. Patients with global aphasia have a poor prognosis and almost never recover completely. Patients with anomic, conduction, and transcortical aphasias have a good prognosis and complete recovery occurs frequently. Patients with Broca's and Wernicke's aphasia have an intermediate prognosis and show a wide range of outcomes. In general, patients with traumatic cases of aphasia do better than those in whom stroke is the cause. Newer techniques of imaging, particularly diffusion-perfusion magnetic resonance imaging, have revealed that many aphasias associated with subcortical infarctions likely result from cortical hypoperfusion and may be reversible with restored perfusion. The bulk of evidence indicates that speech therapy improves the outcome in aphasia. New treatment techniques such as comprehension treatment programs and visual communication therapy are being used to help the patient with aphasia. A team approach to rehabilitation with close cooperation between the neurologist, speech pathologist, and psychologist benefits the patient greatly.

RELATED DISORDERS

1. *Apraxia* is a disturbance of purposeful movement that cannot be accounted for by elementary motor or sensory impairments or by impaired comprehension or cooperation. For example, in dressing apraxia, the patient is unable to dress despite adequate motor power. Apraxias occur commonly in association with aphasic syndromes and usually involve the "disconnection" of one brain area from another.
2. *Agnosias* are disorders of recognition that are not accounted for by elementary perceptual disturbances. For example, visual agnosia is a disorder of recognition not accounted for by a primary disorder of vision. In this condition, the person can see an object but cannot identify it visually. Once the person holds it in his or her hand, he or she usually can identify it by touch.
3. *Gerstmann's syndrome* refers to a lesion of the angular gyrus that causes difficulty writing (agraphia), left–right confusion, difficulty identifying fingers (finger agnosia), and difficulty with calculations (acalculia).

DISCONNECTION SYNDROMES

Disconnection syndromes occur when one part of the cortex is disconnected from the other. Examples include the following:

1. *Alexia without agraphia.* The patient can write but cannot read: lesion in the left occipital region and adjacent corpus callosum. In this syndrome, the preserved right occipital lobe is disconnected from the left-hemisphere language areas.

2. *Balint's syndrome.* The patient has visual inattention and cannot direct gaze to specific points in the visual field despite full extraocular movement (optic ataxia and visual apraxia): bilateral parietooccipital lesions.

3. *Pure word deafness.* The patient cannot interpret words or repeat what is said but can hear sounds and can interpret written language: deep left temporal lobe lesion or bilateral temporal lobe lesions in the primary auditory cortex.

4. *Ideomotor apraxia.* The patient uses left hand well for all functions except those suggested by verbal commands: lesions in left frontal cortex and adjacent corpus callosum.

Suggested Reading

Albert ML. Treatment of aphasia. *Arch Neurol* 1998;55:1417–1419.

Damasio AR. Aphasia. *N Engl J Med* 1992;326:531–539.

Kertesz A. Clinical forms of aphasia. *Acta Neurochir Suppl (Wien)* 1993;56: 52–58.

Pedersen PM, Jorgensen HS, Nakayama H, et al. Aphasia in acute stroke: incidence, determinants, and recovery. *Ann Neurol* 1995;38:659–666.

Saffran EM. Aphasia and the relationship of language and brain. *Semin Neurol* 2000;20(4):409–418.

Chapter 5

Coma

Proper evaluation of the comatose patient involves obtaining a history from family and friends, performing a rapid directed physical and neurologic examination, and obtaining certain laboratory studies while the patient's airway and vital signs are protected. These tasks often are done simultaneously (e.g., one member of the medical team secures the airway, while another talks to the family). An attempt is made to delineate the cause of coma in hopes of finding a treatable process. Treatable causes of coma include metabolic derangements, ingestions, and at times supratentorial processes in the brain (e.g., epidural hematoma). Anatomically, coma implies bilateral hemisphere dysfunction, either structural, drug-induced, or metabolic; unilateral hemisphere disease with compression of the brainstem (e.g., epidural hematoma); or brainstem dysfunction (e.g., pontine hemor-

TABLE 5.1. States of Altered Responsiveness

States of decreased responsiveness
  A. Unresponsive but appears awake
    1. Drowsiness—responds to voice and other stimuli, reduced alertness
    2. Abulic state—frontal lobe disease
    3. Psychiatric diseases—e.g., catatonia
    4. Locked-in syndromes—e.g., pontine infarction
    5. Nonconvulsive status epilepticus
  B. Decreased responsiveness and appears asleep
    1. Stupor—awakens when stimulated but returns to unresponsiveness
    2. Coma—no awakening to stimulation
    3. Psychogenic unresponsiveness

rhage or compression from a posterior fossa mass). If certain basic points are established when examining the comatose patient, the extent of structural central nervous system (CNS) derangement and the cause usually can be determined. One must determine if the patient is comatose or in another state of altered responsiveness (Table 5.1). Comatose patients do not awaken to stimulation of any kind. They may respond with vocalizations, movements, and changes in blood pressure or pulse but do not interact in any meaningful way with the examiner.

ABCs

Before obtaining a history and physical, make sure the patient's *a*irway, *b*reathing, and *c*irculation (ABCs) are stable. Draw blood for glucose, and give 1/2 to 1 amp of 50% dextrose intravenously (IV) (for hypoglycemia). Give thiamine 100 mg IV to avoid precipitating Wernicke's syndrome in patients with alcoholism. This should be given with or before the glucose because glucose alone may precipitate Wernicke's syndrome. Consider naloxone for narcotic ingestion. Then proceed with history, physical, and other diagnostic testing.

Hypoglycemia is one of the most treatable causes of coma.

HISTORY

1. Learn from family or friends whether the patient has a preexisting condition that may explain the coma. Does the patient have diabetes? Is he or she a drug addict or an alcoholic? Does the patient take sleeping pills? Has the patient been depressed? Has the patient sustained recent head trauma? Were there episodes of a similar nature in the past?
2. If a preexisting medical condition exists, is there a factor that may have exacerbated it and precipitated the coma (e.g., chronic liver disease and gastrointestinal bleeding, uremia and infection, a seizure disorder, or failure to take anticonvulsant medication)?
3. A review of all medications, including sleeping pills, and all medical conditions may give hints about the cause of coma.
4. Review the events leading up to the coma. A prodromal febrile illness may suggest meningitis or encephalitis, whereas a despondent patient may suggest the possibility of an overdose.

EXAMINATION

Observe the Patient Carefully

1. Is there *decorticate posturing* (arm flexion with leg extension), implying hemisphere or diencephalon dysfunction that may be caused by destructive lesions or may be secondary to a metabolic derangement?
2. Is there *decerebrate posturing* (extension of legs and arms), implying dysfunction of midbrain or upper pons on a structural or metabolic basis?
3. Is the patient yawning, swallowing, or licking lips? If so, coma cannot be deep and brainstem function is probably intact.
4. Are there repetitive, multifocal, myoclonic jerks (brief muscle twitches in varied muscle groups)? These are characteristic of metabolic encephalopathies, such as hypoxia or uremia. Profound multifocal myoclonus may occur after anoxic injury and implies a poor prognosis.
5. Is there evidence of seizure activity, which sometimes may be as subtle as eye blinking, eye deviation, or facial myoclonus? If so, consider antiepileptic drugs and electroencephalogram (EEG) monitoring. Continued nonconvulsive status may cause irreversible brain injury if not treated.
6. Does the patient only move one side, suggesting a hemiparesis?
7. Are there needle track marks, signs of chronic liver disease, or signs of trauma? Is there a stiff neck, suggesting meningitis? Is the patient poorly groomed and ill appearing, suggesting the possibility of Wernicke's disease?

What Is the Respiratory Pattern?

Cheyne-Stokes respiration (a crescendo–decrescendo breathing pattern with apneic pauses in between) implies bilateral hemisphere dysfunction with an intact brainstem. It often accompanies metabolic disorders and congestive heart failure. Rarely, it may be the first sign of transtentorial herniation.

Central neurogenic hyperventilation (rapid deep breathing) usually indicates damage to the brainstem tegmentum between midbrain and pons.

Apneustic breathing consists of a prolonged inspiratory phase followed by an expiratory pause and usually is seen in pontine infarction.

Ataxic (*irregular or agonal*) breathing is usually a preterminal event signifying disruption of medullary centers.

Remember, significant damage to the brainstem rarely is accompanied by a normal breathing pattern. *Coma with hyperventilation frequently signifies a metabolic derangement:*

Metabolic acidosis: diabetes, uremia, lactic acidosis, poisoning
Respiratory alkalosis: salicylates, hepatic failure
Coma with hypoventilation frequently implies generalized CNS depression secondary to a drug overdose and also occurs in patients with chronic pulmonary disease and CO_2 retention.

Does the Patient Respond to External Stimuli?

1. Apply a noxious stimulus to determine whether the patient is unresponsive. Noxious stimuli may elicit decorticate or decerebrate posturing and, thus, give a clue to the level of brain damage or dysfunction. Movement of only one side is crucial evidence of a hemiparesis caused by brainstem or supratentorial disease. Withdrawal implies purposeful or voluntary behavior.
2. Test for a voluntary response. Are there inconsistencies in the depth of coma? Does the patient avoid noxious stimuli in a directed fashion? Let the patient's hand fall toward the face and see if the patient resists (a check for malingering).
3. Tickling the nose with a cotton swab is a strong noxious stimulus. See if the patient grimaces, opens the eyes, or withdraws the head.
4. Check for a response of the limbs to pain. Is there a low-level reflex, such as flexion, extension, or adduction? Abduction of shoulder or hip usually indicates a higher level (cortical) response.

Examine the Pupils Carefully

Note the size, equality, and light reaction of the pupils.

1. A comatose patient with metabolic intoxication may have no response to external stimuli, absent doll's eyes, and corneal reflexes and yet have intact pupillary responses. Such cases are often secondary to barbiturate ingestion. Remember, reactive pupils in a comatose patient without other responses suggest a metabolic cause.

2. Normal-sized, reactive pupils imply an intact midbrain. Midbrain damage usually produces dilated pupils that do not react to light but may fluctuate in size.

3. Atropine or scopolamine poisoning causes large unreactive pupils that give the false impression of a structural lesion.

4. Pontine damage produces pinpoint pupils that react to bright light when viewed with a magnifying glass. Heroin and pilocarpine also produce pinpoint pupils.

5. A unilaterally fixed, dilated pupil is seen with damage to the third nerve and often is a valuable early sign of a mass effect from a laterally placed supratentorial lesion (see Chapter 31). It also may be caused by direct damage to the midbrain such as by a stroke in the basilar artery territory.

Check Corneal Reflexes and the Doll's Eye Maneuver

Absence of corneal reflexes and doll's eye sign usually means pontine damage or dysfunction. Make sure there is no cervical spine fracture before performing the doll's eye maneuver. Turn the head from side to side to see if the eyes conjugately deviate to the side opposite that to which the head is turned. This may be done in a vertical direction as well. Altered horizontal eye movements usually indicate a pontine lesion, whereas altered vertical eye movements often indicate a midbrain lesion.

If there is no doll's eye response, use ice water irrigation (100–200 mL in each ear), a strong stimulus of the oculovestibular reflex pathway. Be sure that there is no wax in the ears and that the tympanic membranes are intact; check one ear at a time. Tonically deviated eyes to the side of the irrigation (a "normal" brainstem response in a comatose patient) signify that some brainstem function is intact. An intact cortex (e.g., in "coma" caused by hysteria) will cause nystagmus with the fast component opposite to the side of ice water irrigation, as well as nausea and usually significant distress. Absence of the oculovestibular response implies severe depression of brainstem function because it involves a large amount of brainstem territory: cranial nerves III, IV, and VI; the medial longitudinal fasciculus; and the vestibular apparatus.

Motor System Examination Is Important

Hyperreflexia and *up-going* toes or hemiplegia usually mean a structural CNS lesion is the cause of coma. Some exceptions include hepatic coma, hypoglycemia, and uremia, which may be associated with focal signs or hyperreflexia. Nonetheless, these exceptions should be diagnosed quickly by laboratory studies. In hypoxic encephalopathy, the presence of myoclonic status (continuous or recurrent multifocal motor jerks) is indicative of a poor prognosis. *Hyporeflexia* and down-going toes with no hemiplegia generally mean there is no structural CNS lesion, thus indicating drug ingestion or another metabolic cause.

Other Physical Findings

Careful physical examination may detect other clues to the cause of coma (e.g., signs of head trauma in epidural hematoma, barrel chest in pulmonary failure, hepatomegaly in hepatic coma, feeble pulse and hypotension in cardiogenic shock, and stiff neck in meningitis or subarachnoid hemorrhage). There may be cyanosis with hypoxia or "cherry red" appearance in carbon monoxide poisoning. Hypothermia may be associated with barbiturate or ethanol ingestion, whereas hyperthermia may occur in heat stroke.

Laboratory Studies

Laboratory studies must be carried out to exclude metabolic causes of coma such as hypoglycemia, hypercapnia, hypercalcemia, uremia, hepatic failure, electrolyte disturbance, or toxin ingestion. When clinically appropriate, a computed tomography scan is indicated to rule out intracranial hemorrhage (subdural, epidural, or intracerebral), abscess, tumor, or hydrocephalus. An EEG is helpful if seizures are suspected; it is also useful for metabolic encephalopathy (slowing and triphasic waves) or for psychogenic coma (normal EEG). A lumbar puncture may be needed to detect infection or subarachnoid hemorrhage, although one must be certain that there is no shift of midline structures before the lumbar puncture. Other therapeutic measures, such as treatment of increased intracranial pressure or gastric lavage after ingestions, may be required. Remember, for a patient with coma, the neurologic examination should define whether a diffuse disorder, structural supratentorial disease, or infratentorial disease is most likely. The history and general examination provide clues to the etiology of coma.

Note: A discussion of the approach to the patient who is "brain dead" or who is thought to be in "irreversible coma" is beyond the scope of this manual (see Suggested Reading). Principles found useful for house officers when approaching the latter problems include the following: (a) obtaining appropriate consultations and tests (e.g., nuclear medicine brain scan) before major therapeutic decisions are made; (b) paying meticulous attention to good communication between all members of the health care team and with family members; and (c) identifying one physician (usually the admitting physician or primary treating physician) who assumes the primary responsibility for collating the clinical information, consulting with the family, and making the major therapeutic decisions. There are usually "brain death" criteria published at each hospital.

Suggested Reading

American Neurological Association Committee on Ethical Affairs. Persistent vegetative state. *Ann Neurol* 1993;33:386–390.

Chiappa KH, Hill RA. Evaluation and prognostication in coma. *Electroencephalogr Clin Neurophysiol* 1998;106:149–155.

Edgren E, Kelsey S, Sutton-Tyrell K, et al. Assessment of neurological prognosis in comatose survivors of cardiac arrest. *Lancet* 1994;343: 1055–1059.

Feske SK. Coma and confusional states: emergency diagnosis and management. *Neurol Clin* 1998;16:237–256.

Hamel MB, Goldman L, Teno J, et al. Identification of comatose patients at high risk for death or severe disability. *JAMA* 1995;273:1842–1848.

Liu GT. Coma. *Neurosurg Clin North Am* 1999;10:579–586.

Madl C, Kramer L, Yeganehfar W, et al. Detection of nontraumatic comatose patients with no benefit of intensive care treatment by recording of sensory evoked potentials. *Arch Neurol* 1996;53: 512–516.

Multi-Society Task Force on PVS. Medical aspects of the persistent vegetative state. *N Engl J Med* 1994;330:1572–1579.

Ropper AH. Lateral displacement of the brain and level of consciousness in patients with an acute hemispheral mass. *N Engl J Med* 1986;314: 953–960.

Samuels MA. The evaluation of comatose patients. *Hosp Pract* 1993;28: 165–182.

Wijdicks EFM. Determining brain death in adults. *Neurology* 1995;45: 1003–1011.

Widjicks EFM, Parisi JE, Sharbrough FW. Prognostic value of myoclonus status in comatose survivors of cardiac arrest. *Ann Neurol* 1994;35: 239–245.

Chapter 6

Vertigo-Dizziness

Vertigo implies the illusory sensation of turning or spinning—either of the patients themselves or of their environment. *Dizziness* is a nonspecific term and may be used by the patient to describe a variety of sensations such as lightheadedness, spinning, or a feeling of instability. Although vertigo may be distinguished from dizziness by demanding that unmistakable whirling or turning be present, these two symptoms overlap clinically and may be approached as one entity.

IS THE PROCESS PERIPHERAL, CENTRAL, OR SYSTEMIC?

The goal of the clinician is to decide whether the cause is *peripheral* (labyrinth, vestibular, or cochlear nerve), *central* (brainstem, cerebellum, or cerebral cortex), or *systemic* (e.g., cardiovascular, metabolic). A careful history is often helpful in making the distinction.

HISTORY

Can the Dizziness Be Better Defined?

When the patient describes dizziness, ask that the sensation be better defined. Is the patient really feeling lightheaded—a feeling that he or she may pass out, with visual blurring and a sense that the surrounding world is far away? That implies a reduction in perfusion to the brain as a mechanism. Or is the patient having vertigo (a sensation of spinning)? This implies a disorder of the vestibular system and its central connections. Is the patient feeling unsteady but not vertiginous? This implies a disorder of balance, sensory perception, or visual impairment. Ask the patient to use other words than "dizziness" to describe the feeling being experienced.

Questions to Ask

1. Are the symptoms paroxysmal, and are they related to head position or other precipitating factors? (Vertigo often is worsened with changes in head position.)
2. Is there associated nausea, vomiting, or headache? (These may be seen with migraine or intracranial processes.)
3. Are symptoms of diplopia, dysarthria, or numbness present? (This suggests a brainstem lesion.)
4. Is there tinnitus or deafness? (These suggest eighth nerve or ear involvement.)
5. Is there a lapse of awareness? (This suggests seizures or syncope.)
6. Does the event occur on standing or after arising? (This suggests syncope or presyncope.)
7. Are there palpitations? (This suggests a cardiac cause.)
8. Does the patient describe a sense of unsteadiness? (This suggests a balance disorder.)
9. Is the patient taking many medications, or does the patient have a psychiatric history? (Medications may cause nonspecific dizziness or vertigo. Patients with anxiety or hyperventilation may describe dizziness.)

EXAMINATION OF THE PATIENT

1. A general *physical* examination should include careful attention to the cardiovascular system. Is there postural hypotension? Does the patient have an arrhythmia?
2. Specifically check the ear canal and hearing (listening to a watch tick, the spoken voice, and finger-rubbing screens three basic frequencies).
3. Perform a complete neurologic examination with special attention to cranial nerves, coordination, and the presence of nystagmus (horizontal, vertical, or rotatory).
4. Check for positional vertigo and nystagmus by having the patient go from a sitting to a supine position while quickly

turning the head to the side and with the neck extended 30 degrees. Note nystagmus, latency of the response, associated vertigo, and fatigability of the response.

5. Caloric testing (minimal ice water caloric test) may be performed. Patient lies supine with the head elevated 30 degrees. Irrigate each ear with 0.2 mL ice water (tuberculin syringe). Notice any asymmetry between the response in each ear.

6. Consider having the patient hyperventilate for 1 to 2 minutes. Patients with hyperventilation syndrome rapidly reproduce their symptoms, often with paresthesias of the limbs and around the mouth, soon after starting this maneuver.

IS THE LESION PERIPHERAL OR CENTRAL IN ORIGIN?

With vertigo, a major goal of the clinician is to decide whether the lesion is *peripheral* (labyrinth, vestibular, or cochlear nerve) or *central* (brainstem, cerebellum, or cerebral cortex). A careful history is often helpful in making this distinction.

Peripheral lesions causing vertigo may be associated with deafness and tinnitus (signs of eighth nerve dysfunction); there are no central signs. If caloric testing reproduces the patient's dizziness or there is a unilaterally decreased caloric response, the lesion is usually peripheral. Central lesions are defined by central nervous system (CNS) signs or symptoms (e.g., ataxia, cranial nerve abnormalities, diplopia, dysarthria, papilledema). Vertigo of peripheral origin tends to parallel the severity of the nystagmus. In central lesions, there is often marked nystagmus with little or no vertigo; the nystagmus is most prominent when looking toward the side of the lesion, and the fast component of the nystagmus usually changes with looking in different directions. In acute labyrinthine and vestibular nerve disorders, the nystagmus is usually more prominent when looking toward the good ear. In peripheral vestibulopathy, the patient falls toward the side of the lesion and away from the fast component of nystagmus. In central lesions such as cerebellar infarction, the patient falls toward the side of the lesion and toward the fast component of nystagmus. *Vertical nystagmus* is a sign of brainstem disease unless the patient is taking medication (especially barbiturates). *Rotary or torsional nystagmus* generally is seen with peripheral lesions.

TABLE 6.1. Differentiation of Peripheral versus Central Nystagmus

	Peripheral	Central
Latency	3–10 seconds	None
Fatigability	Yes	No
Associated symptoms	Nausea, vomiting	Diplopia, dysarthria
Vertical nystagmus	Absent	May be present
Rotatory nystagmus	Common	Uncommon

Test for Positional Nystagmus

Testing for positional nystagmus may be helpful in discriminating peripheral from central vertigo. The Barany maneuver is used. The patient is taken from a sitting position to lying flat with the head extended over the edge of the bed 30 degrees, with the head turned to the left or the right. Positional nystagmus of peripheral origin usually begins 3 to 10 seconds after assuming the new head position (latency of the response), is commonly associated with vertigo and nausea, lasts up to 10 seconds, and is fatigable (it becomes harder to elicit the nystagmus after several consecutive tries) (Table 6.1). *Positional nystagmus of central origin* begins immediately, may last longer than 10 seconds, and is not fatigable; nausea and vertigo are not prominent.

IS THE LESION PERIPHERAL?

Middle ear disease may affect the labyrinth. Check for otitis or a history of recent ear infection and other abnormalities of the tympanic membrane. Establish whether the patient has been exposed to ototoxic drugs. Remember, excessive wax in the ear can cause dizziness. Symptoms related to middle ear disease may be brought out by pressure applied to the external ear.

Ménière's disease is a recurrent disease with a characteristic triad: episodic vertigo, tinnitus, and deafness. The underlying mechanism probably relates to swelling of the endolymphatic space. Before vertigo appears there may be a buildup with tinnitus and "stuffiness"; the attack is violent and includes nausea, vomiting, sweating, and decreased hearing. Patients often note a "full" feeling on the side of the affected ear. Nystagmus is present only during the attack, and the direction may vary. Ménière's disease occurs in patients from the ages of 30 to 60 years and is accompanied by residual tinnitus and hearing loss after multiple attacks. The vertigo is sudden, recurrent, and severe; it usually lasts 1 to 2 hours, not seconds or days. Treatment includes bed rest, sedatives, fluids, antihistamines, and antiemetics during the attack; prophylactically, some use diuretics and sodium restriction. Surgical therapy (endolymphatic shunt) is recommended in some chronic cases.

Benign paroxysmal positional vertigo (BPPV) occurs when the patient turns the head or changes position; it can be reproduced by testing for positional nystagmus. There is no hearing loss, calorics are normal, and the disorder may be self-limited. Treatment with meclizine is usually beneficial if the symptoms are acute. In patients with chronic BPPV, a variety of exercises may terminate the symptoms by moving otolithic particles away from the affected portion of the inner ear where they are altering movements of the labyrinthine hair cells. The patient should avoid sudden changes in head position.

Acute labyrinthitis may be secondary to bacterial or viral infections. The onset may be sudden, with severe vertigo and gastrointestinal symptoms. The attack lasts 1 to 3 days. There usually is spontaneous nystagmus toward the good ear, hearing may or may not be affected, and calorics are usually normal. Treatment is symptomatic (i.e., bed rest plus meclizine or lorazepam).

Vestibular neuronitis refers to sudden attacks of vertigo and nausea with no auditory signs or symptoms. Caloric testing shows hypofunction of the affected side, which serves to distinguish it from labyrinthitis. Treatment is symptomatic.

Geniculate ganglionitis causes vertigo associated with ear pain and facial paralysis. It may be caused by herpes zoster infection (Ramsay Hunt syndrome). Look for periauricular herpes eruption.

Posttraumatic vertigo is common, and damage to the labyrinth is the postulated mechanism because symptoms are those of peripheral vestibulopathy. The prognosis is good, with symptoms subsiding over a period of weeks.

DOES THE LESION BEGIN PERIPHERALLY THEN SPREAD CENTRALLY?

Acoustic neuroma begins from sheath cells of the vestibular portion of the eighth nerve in the internal auditory canal; thus tinnitus, decreased hearing (e.g., trouble hearing on the phone), and dizziness or disequilibrium are early complaints. As the tumor grows in to the cerebellopontine angle, cranial nerve dysfunction (loss of corneal reflex, facial weakness) and cerebellar signs become prominent. Diagnosis is not difficult once there is obvious CNS involvement. Because such tumors can be small and confined to the internal auditory canal, a contrast-enhanced magnetic resonance imaging (MRI) is the imaging modality of choice. Brainstem auditory evoked response is a sensitive screening tool for acoustic neuroma. Early recognition depends on considering the diagnosis in patients with dizziness, unsteadiness, or symptoms referable to the eighth nerve (tinnitus and decreased hearing).

IS THE LESION CENTRAL?

Posterior fossa tumors may cause vertigo or dizziness; look for cerebellar and other brainstem signs. Check for evidence of increased intracranial pressure in patients with vertigo and headache by examination of the fundi.

Vascular disease (vertebrobasilar insufficiency) may cause vertigo. To establish that vertebrobasilar insufficiency is the cause, note other brainstem symptoms (diplopia, slurred speech, numbness, trouble swallowing) or signs (cranial nerve dysfunction, motor or sensory loss). Other important points include the following:

1. Dizziness or vertigo alone may be the *first* sign of vertebrobasilar insufficiency, but most patients have accompanying signs or symptoms of brainstem dysfunction.
2. The *lateral medullary syndrome* (Chapter 16) may begin with vertigo.
3. *Cerebellar hemorrhage or infarction* may begin with the acute onset of dizziness, vomiting, inability to walk or stand, and severe headache (see Chapter 16).
4. If dizziness is accompanied by *eighth nerve dysfunction* only, it is probably not vascular in origin.
5. Vertigo is seldom a feature of carotid artery disease.

Temporal lobe epilepsy is an important cause of dizziness and vertigo. Note a history of staring spells, automatisms, déjà vu, or abdominal pain. Workup for this seizure disorder should include a sleep electroencephalogram. Effective treatment is available (antiepileptic drugs).

Basilar migraine may be associated with vertigo and is characterized by symptoms in the basilar artery territory. Check for vertigo, visual disturbances (including scotomata), tinnitus, blackouts, and associated complaints of throbbing occipital headache. It usually occurs in young females. Treatment includes prophylactic migraine medication. Patients with migraine have a higher frequency of vertigo or dizziness than the general population.

Dizziness after *head trauma* may be the result of eighth nerve injury, benign paroxysmal vertigo, or represent posttraumatic epilepsy.

Check for a history of *diplopia*. Acute difficulty with eye movements may result in dizziness or vertigo. *Multiple sclerosis* may present with dizziness or diplopia as a result of brainstem involvement (see Chapter 21).

IS THE LESION SYSTEMIC?

Important causes to consider are cardiac arrhythmias, hypertension or hypotension, congestive heart failure, anemia, hypoglycemia, thyroid disease, and a variety of drugs (e.g., ototoxic drugs, especially the aminoglycosides, antihypertensives, salicylates). Patients with multiple sensory deficits (e.g., poor vision and neuropathy) may complain of dizziness. (This is seen most commonly in the elderly.)

LABORATORY EVALUATION

Laboratory studies that may prove useful in the evaluation of the patient with vertigo or dizziness include the following: (a) brainstem auditory evoked responses, particularly sensitive for acoustic neuromas; (b) electronystagmography, particularly sensitive for peripheral labyrinthopathies; and (c) MRI for structural lesions of the posterior fossa and eighth nerve and cochlea. The history and physical examination are more important than laboratory testing in patients with "dizziness."

DIZZINESS OR VERTIGO WITH NO APPARENT CAUSE

Vertigo can be caused by psychogenic factors or by hyperventilation. In a study of a large series of patients who complained of dizziness, one of the most common causes was hyperventilation. Patients with somatoform disorders and phobias also may complain of dizziness. Occasionally, despite careful evaluation, a patient's dizziness appears to be idiopathic. In these circumstances, symptomatic treatment and careful follow-up of the patient are required.

TREATMENT

Drugs that may be useful in the treatment of dizziness or vertigo include meclizine, other antihistamines, diazepam or lorazepam, and anticholinergics. The patient also should be advised to avoid sudden positional changes. Limiting intake of caffeine, nicotine, alcohol, and salt may be of benefit. In some cases of severe incapacitating vertigo, surgery (such as closure of an endolymphatic fistula) is necessary. Recent studies have emphasized the importance of the diagnosis and treatment of BPPV. Specific maneuvers to treat BPPV are available and are effective. A graded series of exercises may be helpful in other patients with chronic vertigo of peripheral or central origin. Antiepileptic drugs are useful in the rare patient who has vertigo as a manifestation of simple partial seizures.

Suggested Reading

Brandt T, Steddin S, Daroff RB. Therapy for benign paroxysmal positioning vertigo, revisited. *Neurology* 1994;44:796–800.

Brown JJ. A systematic approach to the dizzy patient. *Neurol Clin* 1990;8: 209–224.

Cutrer FM, Baloh RW. Migraine-associated dizziness. *Headache* 1992;32: 300–304.

Gizzi M, Riley E, Molinari S. The diagnostic value of imaging the patient with dizziness. *Arch Neurol* 1996;53:1299–1304.

Hain TC. Treatment of vertigo. *Neurologist* 1995;1:125–133.

Hotson J, Baloh RW. The acute vestibular syndrome. *N Engl J Med* 1998; 339:680–685

Knox GW, McPherson A. Meniere's disease: differential diagnosis and treatment. *Am Fam Physician* 1997;55:1185–1190, 1193–1194.

Slattery WH, Fayad JN. Medical treatment of Meniere's disease. *Otolaryngol Clin North Am* 1997;30:1027–1037.

Sloane PD. Evaluation and management of dizziness in the older patient. *Clin Geriatr Med* 1996;12:785–801.

Chapter 7

Hyperreflexia

Normal reflexes suggest that the motor system is functioning appropriately. The main motor pathway, the corticospinal tract, descends from the cortex to different segments of the spinal cord. Neurons in this tract are upper motor neurons, and the tract is also known as the pyramidal tract. These neurons synapse with lower motor neurons in the anterior grey matter of the spinal cord at the root level where the lower motor neuron exits. The corticospinal tract travels from the motor cortex through the internal capsule and down the cerebral peduncles in the midbrain; it then crosses in the pyramids of the medulla and follows the lateral corticospinal tract in the spinal cord. Pathologically hyperactive reflexes imply disease in the corticospinal tract, an upper motor neuron disorder. Other signs of upper motor neuron disorder include spasticity, clonus, slow motor movements, and weakness of certain muscle groups (deltoid, triceps, wrist and finger extensors, hip flexors, knee flexors, and ankle dorsiflexors and evertors.). An up-going toe (a positive Babinski sign) is a cardinal manifestation of upper motor neuron dysfunction. In the acute phase of an upper motor neuron lesion, hyporeflexia often is present, with hyperreflexia slowly developing over 1 to 2 weeks.

Many people have exaggerated reflexes. A good rule is that symmetrically hyperactive reflexes with down-going toes are usually normal. Significant upper motor neuron dysfunction usually is accompanied by up-going toes. An exception to this rule is if there is a concurrent lower motor neuron weakness of the toe extensors, so that the toe cannot go up. Superficial abdominal reflexes (stroking the skin next to the umbilicus elicits reflex movement of that part of the abdominal wall) may be absent on the side of pyramidal tract dysfunction. A brisk jaw jerk in patients with hyperreflexia suggests bilateral lesions above the mid-pons.

UNILATERAL HYPERREFLEXIA

Unilateral hyperreflexia or a unilateral up-going toe implies upper motor neuron injury on one side of the nervous system (same side of the spinal cord or the opposite side of brainstem, internal capsule, or cortex). Decide whether this represents an old lesion that does not require further investigation or a newly developing one. You will need to check for the following:

1. *History of birth injury.* An otherwise normal person may have unilateral hyperreflexia with no apparent cause. The unilateral hyperreflexia may be a result of birth injury with mild cerebral palsy.
2. *Old neurologic disease.* A patient with a history of meningitis, stroke, subdural hematoma, or the like may have unilateral hyperreflexia. Remember, a small stroke may not have been recognized by the patient.
3. *Asymptomatic cervical cord disease.* This disease may cause unilateral hyperreflexia in older people.
4. *Newly developing signs or symptoms.* If history suggests this, a full investigation is warranted.

Note: Unilateral corticospinal tract signs may be subtle. Look for a mild pronator drift, slowing of fine motor movements on one side, a tendency to flex the arm while walking, and the inability to roll the arms alternately around each other. In a unilateral disorder, the good arm may roll around the paretic arm.

BILATERAL HYPERREFLEXIA

Bilateral hyperreflexia with up-going toes implies bilateral pyramidal tract dysfunction. Note the following:

1. Consider *spinal cord compression* as a cause. Ask about a sensory loss, bowel and bladder dysfunction, back pain, or weakness in the legs. Check for a sensory level, motor level,

local back tenderness or deformity, or a lax sphincter (see Chapter 9).

2. *Cervical spondylosis* is the most common cause of spinal cord dysfunction in the elderly. Ask about neck pain, weakness, or paresthesias in the arms. Check for hyperreflexia, muscle wasting in the arms, radicular sensory changes in the arms, decreased range of motion of the neck, and degenerative changes on radiograph of the cervical spine.

3. *Multiple sclerosis* (MS) is an important cause of hyperreflexia in young and middle-aged patients. Establish whether there are "multiple lesions in time and space." If MS is suspected, obtain brain magnetic resonance imaging (see Chapter 21).

4. *Multiple small strokes* (état lacunaire) can cause bilateral hyperreflexia and frequently are seen in the elderly with hypertension or diabetes. Check for a history of multiple small strokes (although they may have been clinically silent) and for other evidence of vascular disease (e.g., bruits, decreased peripheral pulses). Search for other signs of "multiple stroke" syndrome: emotional lability, brisk jaw jerk, increased gag reflex, and ataxia (features of pseudobulbar palsy). In addition, there usually is a concurrent dementia with memory impairment.

5. *Familial spastic paraparesis* may present with slowly progressive bilateral hyperreflexia and spasticity. Check for a family history and high arched feet. Leukodystrophies may have similar signs. Human T-lymphotropic virus type 1 (HTLV-I) infection also may cause spastic paraparesis.

6. *Metabolic causes of hyperreflexia* include hepatic and uremic encephalopathy, B_{12} deficiency, and adrenoleukodystrophies.

7. *Amyotrophic lateral sclerosis* (ALS) causes increased reflexes caused by pyramidal tract involvement in the brainstem or spinal cord. Brainstem (corticobulbar) involvement causes brisk jaw jerk, hyperactive gag reflex, dysarthria, and dysphagia. In addition, anterior horn cell (lower motor neuron) involvement causes fasciculations, wasting, and weakness often most prominent in the arms. The combination of upper and lower motor neuron signs in spinal cord and brainstem without sensory loss is virtually diagnostic of ALS, particularly with bulbar or pseudobulbar involvement.

8. Hyperreflexia can be seen in otherwise normal, anxious patients.

HYPERREFLEXIA IN THE LEGS ONLY

Hyperreflexia in both arms and legs implies a lesion at the cervical cord or higher; *hyperreflexia in the legs* implies a lesion below the cervical cord. Lesions in the thoracic cord include tumors, disc protrusions, trauma, and vascular malformations. Sometimes hyperreflexia occurs in the legs from lesions above the thoracic region.

1. In *cerebral palsy,* leg fibers may be selectively involved in the white matter of the hemispheres, giving increased reflexes in the legs only ("spastic diparesis").
2. *Cervical spinal stenosis* may present with only leg weakness and spasticity, with relatively few symptoms of arm or neck involvement.
3. By virtue of their location, *parasagittal intracranial masses* may affect cortical leg fibers producing hyperreflexia in legs only, mimicking a cord lesion. Headache, seizures, papilledema, or personality change may be present.
4. *Hydrocephalus* may present with spastic paraparesis because parasagittal leg fibers are stretched most by dilated lateral ventricles.
5. *Arnold-Chiari malformation* with cerebellar tonsillar ectopia and brainstem deformity may be associated with a spastic paraparesis.

Suggested Reading

Adams RD, Victor M, Ropper AH. *Disorders of motility. Principles of neurology.* New York: McGraw-Hill, 1997;45–63.

Chapter 8

Hyporeflexia/Peripheral Neuropathy

Hypoactive reflexes are caused by disease between the spinal cord and muscle, typically involving the root, plexus, or peripheral nerves. One component of the reflex pathway is abnormal: peripheral nerve, sensory root, anterior horn cells in cord, motor roots, or muscle. Disturbances of any part of the reflex arc may cause hyporeflexia. Reflexes can be reinforced by having patients pull their hands apart or bite down while the reflex is tested. Patients voluntarily tensing their muscles will diminish or extinguish the reflex and may need to be distracted. Areflexia implies no reflexes, even with reinforcement; reflexes present only with reinforcement imply an intact reflex pathway and may or may not be abnormal. Consider the following points when confronted with hyporeflexia:

1. *Normally hypoactive reflexes.* Occasionally, normal individuals may have hyporeflexia with no other obvious cause. The presence of a reflex with reinforcement and absence of other signs are reassuring.
2. *Delayed relaxation phase of the reflex.* This unique hypoactive or "hung up" reflex is classic for hypothyroidism and at times serves as the first clue to this metabolic abnormality. It is best seen in the ankle jerk reflex.
3. *Spinal shock.* This is an important cause of areflexia and often is seen during the initial stages of cord damage—whether traumatic, vascular, or neoplastic in origin. Although compressive damage to spinal cord generally causes hyperactive reflexes, remember that acutely (during the first days and

often as long as 1 to 2 weeks) reflexes may be depressed or absent. Be sure to check for a sensory level, especially if there is leg weakness.

4. *Acute stroke.* Initially, there may be hyporeflexia on the side of the hemiparesis; hyperreflexia usually develops within a few days.

5. *Asymptomatic areflexia with a large pupil.* This is a benign syndrome (Adie's syndrome) consisting of generalized areflexia with a large pupil that reacts to accommodation but only slowly to direct light.

6. *Myopathy.* Muscle disorders may cause hyporeflexia but usually not areflexia. The decrease in reflex is consistent with the degree of muscle wasting and weakness. Remember, weakness from muscle disease is generally more marked proximally (shoulder and hip), whereas weakness from peripheral nerve disease is more marked distally (hand and foot). Neuromuscular junction disorders usually spare the reflexes.

7. *Isolated unilaterally absent reflex.* This important sign of disc disease compressing spinal roots can be seen with diseases affecting specific peripheral nerves. Some examples are as follows:

   ■ *Unilaterally absent ankle jerk* should arouse suspicion of disk disease with compression of the S1 root on the same side. (Ask the patient about sciatic pain, and check straight leg raising.) Similarly, but less frequently, the knee jerk may be absent unilaterally with root disease at L3 or L4 or with femoral neuropathy (see Chapter 10).

   ■ *Unilaterally absent brachioradialis, biceps, or triceps* reflex may imply impingement on C5, C6, or C7 nerve roots, respectively, in the cervical region from cervical spondylosis.

   ■ Remember, *mononeuropathy and plexus injuries,* whether traumatic or from tumor, are other important causes of asymmetric reflex loss (see Chapter 10).

8. *Bilateral areflexia* is a key sign of neuropathy (discussed later). A patient with no reflexes usually has a neuropathy.

PERIPHERAL NEUROPATHY

Peripheral neuropathies occur in a broad category of diseases, many of which are common and treatable. The key manifestations include bilateral or multifocal hyporeflexia, sensory or motor involvement, and (at times) autonomic dysfunction.

Peripheral neuropathies are characterized in a variety of ways, which may help in establishing their etiology. The temporal profile may be acute, subacute, or chronic. The pattern may be distal or proximal, symmetric or asymmetric, diffuse or multifocal. The nerve fibers involved may be sensory, motor, autonomic, or a combination thereof. The pathology may be axonal (involving the nerve itself), demyelinating (involving the nerve sheath), or a combination. It may be vasculitic (inflammation to the blood vessels supplying the nerve causing nerve injury) or neuronal (involving the cell body). The fiber type involved may preferentially be large fiber (vibration and position sense impairment with sparing of pin, temperature, and autonomic fibers) or small fiber (selective pin, temperature, and autonomic involvement).

The history and physical examination often help to establish possible etiologies. For example, a rapidly progressive course with areflexia, vibration loss, and proximal and distal weakness occurring after a viral illness suggests an acute demyelinating inflammatory polyneuropathy. A slow course, distal muscle wasting in the feet, distal pin and vibration loss, and loss of ankle jerks suggest a chronic, axonal sensorimotor polyneuropathy.

Acute Areflexia with Weakness

1. *Acute areflexia, with weakness and little sensory loss.* This is the classic presentation of acute inflammatory demyelinating polyneuropathy (AIDP), or *Guillain-Barré syndrome.* This may follow a systemic infection or vaccination by days or weeks, or it may occur after an event such as a surgery.

   a. *Clinical characteristics.* It is typical to have progressive weakness over a few days, with gait unsteadiness, arm weakness, and facial and respiratory involvement, sometimes with an "ascending" pattern. In *mild* forms, the patient's motor difficulties are confined to problems with gait and difficulty using the upper extremities. The dysfunction does not progress, and a clue to the diagnosis is the areflexia. With severe weakness, ventilatory assistance may be necessary. A form in which cranial nerve involvement predominates is called the Miller-Fisher variant (characterized by ophthalmoparesis, ataxia, and areflexia). Autonomic dysfunction may occur, causing bladder dysfunction and fluctuations of blood pressure, heart rate, and temperature. Usually, the disease is monophasic and patients recover, although the recovery may take months in severely affected patients.

b. *Diagnosis.* Clinical features include rapidly progressive muscle weakness of proximal and distal muscles, areflexia, mild distal sensory loss, and bifacial weakness (an important clue). Cerebrospinal fluid (CSF) initially may be normal, but over days it shows an increase in protein with few or no white cells. Nerve conduction studies also may be normal initially, but they ultimately show evidence of a demyelinating polyneuropathy.

c. *Treatment.* Because of the potential for respiratory failure and dangerous autonomic fluctuations, careful monitoring of respiratory and cardiac function is mandatory once the diagnosis is made. Vital capacity and negative inspiratory force are useful in studying respiratory function and predicting the need for ventilator assistance. Treatment to avoid decubiti, pressure palsies, deep vein thrombosis, and other intensive care unit (ICU) complications is important. Plasmapheresis has been shown in large randomized studies to shorten the duration of illness, especially ICU course and time in hospital. This is most useful if begun within the first week of the disease. Intravenous gamma globulin (IVIG) may be of equal benefit. Unless severe axonal injury occurs, a complete or near-complete recovery is expected in weeks or months.

d. *Differential diagnosis.* Other causes of acute symmetric motor weakness that may mimic AIDP include acute intermittent porphyria, tick paralysis, Lyme disease, acquired immunodeficiency virus (AIDS), botulism, toxin exposure, diphtheria (palatal and extraocular muscle palsies), and polyarteritis. Think of polio in unimmunized children. Consider mononucleosis, hepatitis, and *Mycoplasma* as preceding infections that triggered the illness. A slower course or a relapsing picture suggests chronic inflammatory demyelinating polyneuropathy (CIDP), which is treated with prednisone or IVIG.

2. *Areflexia with sensory involvement* and little or late developing motor loss. A variety of systemic illnesses may cause predominantly a sensory neuropathy that may progress over weeks to years. Consider the following:

a. *Diabetes.* Various neuropathies may be associated with diabetes (see Chapter 22); most common is a bilateral symmetric neuropathy manifested by absent ankle jerks and decreased vibration sense. Motor weakness is minimal.

b. *Alcoholism* (neuropathy is the result of a nutritional deficit). These patients have a sensory neuropathy, often painful, involving feet and hands, including decreased vibration sense (see Chapter 27). They complain of numbness and tingling, and their feet are tender to touch. Weakness is minimal, although this distal sensory neuropathy occasionally progresses to an incapacitating motor neuropathy.

c. *Vitamin B_{12} deficiency.* This may cause a sensory neuropathy often associated with spinal cord involvement. Characteristic findings include loss of vibration and position sense, distal reflex loss and paresthesias, and up-going toes.

d. *Medications.* Cisplatinum and other medications may cause a predominantly sensory neuropathy.

e. *Uremia.* Patients with uremia may have sensory or sensorimotor involvement with "restless" leg symptoms and burning paresthesias (see Chapter 26).

f. *Malignancy.* A malignancy (especially lung cancer) may have a sensory neuropathy as the presenting complaint as part of a paraneoplastic syndrome

g. *Amyloidosis.* This disease, either primary or secondary to another systemic illness, may cause a sensory and autonomic neuropathy, preferentially affecting small fibers (pain, temperature, sweating loss, trophic changes).

h. *Sjögren's syndrome.* This common and underrecognized rheumatologic condition may be associated with a predominantly sensory syndrome of ataxia, limb involvement, and subacute to chronic course. Ask about dry eyes, dry mouth, and arthritic symptoms.

i. *Note:* A familial sensory radicular neuropathy with autosomal dominant inheritance may present during the second and third decades. Fabry's and Refsum's diseases may present as sensory neuropathy.

3. *A multifocal pattern with asymmetric motor and sensory involvement.* This pattern may be seen with demyelinating neuropathies and with vasculitic neuropathies. Vasculitis, diabetes, sarcoidosis Lyme disease, leprosy, and AIDS are disorders to consider. Tomaculous neuropathy is a familial disorder with multiple compression palsies (i.e., median at the wrist, ulnar at the elbow, peroneal at the knee).

4. *Chronic, distal, relatively symmetric motor and sensory neuropathy.* This is the most common pattern of neuropathy. Often it is caused by diabetes mellitus and is seen with many other systemic disorders such as nutritional deficits, toxins, uremia, hypothyroidism, dysproteinemias, collagen vascular diseases, and paraneoplastic conditions.

5. *Bilateral areflexia and neuropathy on a familial basis.* The prototype for familial neuropathy is *Charcot-Marie-Tooth* disease (peroneal muscular atrophy). These patients have sensory loss, "champagne-bottle" legs, a widespread areflexia not merely confined to the ankles, and pes cavus. Familial neuropathies may be associated with other inherited neurologic diseases and accompanied by other signs (i.e., tremor, nystagmus, optic atrophy, etc.).

6. *Predominantly motor neuropathy.* Amyotrophic lateral sclerosis is the archetype; however, some paraneoplastic and toxic neuropathies also may be predominantly motor. Check for antibodies to GM1 and MAG. Porphyria may present as an acute motor neuropathy. Nerve conduction studies will help define those that spare the sensory fibers.

7. *Autonomic neuropathy.* This may be seen with diabetes or alcoholism or as a paraneoplastic syndrome, and it may occur with toxins and amyloidosis. An acute autonomic neuropathy also has been described as a postinfectious complication. Familial autonomic neuropathies include Riley-Day syndrome. Symptoms include orthostatic hypotension, sweating abnormalities, gastrointestinal (GI) symptoms, impotence, and bladder dysfunction. Check for orthostatic hypotension and measure the cardiac R-R interval from a rhythm strip.

WORKUP OF NEUROPATHIES

In some cases, the clinical history and examination will define the etiology of the neuropathy without extensive investigation. In other instances, a directed workup, keeping in mind the type of neuropathy and possible etiologies, is required for a diagnosis. In some instances, no diagnosis emerges despite extensive workup (most commonly in chronic distal sensorimotor axonal neuropathies).

Check these important points when dealing with a neuropathic process of undetermined cause:

1. Is there evidence of toxin exposure (painful red feet; GI disturbances), such as thallium (alopecia), lead (affects upper extremities, including motor neuropathies with wristdrop, and causes lead line in gums), or other metals (copper, zinc, mercury)? Consider organic toxins and occupational exposures.

2. Check for drugs that may cause neuropathy. Nitrofurantoin, isoniazid, vincristine, and cisplatinum are common offenders. Look up each medication and any "herbal" medications that the patient takes.

3. Does the patient have an associated systemic illness: hypothyroidism, syphilis, amyloid (large tongue, GI symptoms), myeloma or other gammopathy, leprosy (anesthetic skin patches), lupus, AIDS, Lyme disease, sarcoid, polyarteritis, pernicious anemia, porphyria, diabetes, renal failure, polyarteritis, rheumatoid arthritis, Sjögren's syndrome, or systemic sclerosis?

4. Is the neuropathy relapsing? CIDP, alcohol, lead, or porphyria may be the cause.

5. Electromyography and nerve conduction studies assist in establishing the presence of neuropathy (characterizing the pattern as predominantly axonal, demyelinating, or multifocal; motor or sensory; large fiber or small fiber) and may give clues to possible etiologies.

6. Nerve biopsy is useful only in a small group of patients and, in many cases, is nonspecific. It is most beneficial when considering a demyelinating neuropathy, vasculitis, amyloidosis, or sarcoid.

7. Spinal fluid is usually nondiagnostic but may show increased protein in inflammatory neuropathies, diabetes, and neu-

ropathies associated with cancer. Any neuropathy affecting
the proximal root may increase CSF protein.

TREATMENT OF NEUROPATHIES

Treatment depends on the etiology, removal of the offending
toxin or drug, treatment of the underlying systemic illness, or
treatment of a specific remediable neuropathy. Vitamin supplementation may be helpful, particularly in nutritional neuropathies. Immunosuppression may be useful in immunologically
mediated neuropathies. Rehabilitative devices and avoidance of
pressure palsies is helpful in some neuropathies. The treatment
of painful neuropathies is reviewed in Chapter 29.

Note: A mnemonic device that may aid in remembering
causes of neuropathy is "DANG THERAPIST": **D**iabetes, **A**lcohol,
Nutritional, **G**uillain-Barré, **T**oxins, **HE**reditary, **R**efsum's, **A**my-
loid, **P**orphyria, **I**nfection, **S**ystemic, and **T**umor.

Suggested Reading

Chalk CH. Acquired peripheral neuropathy. *Neurol Clin* 1997;15:
    501–528.
Dyck PJ, Dyck JB, Chalk CH. The 10 P's: a mnemonic helpful in charac-
    terization and differential diagnosis of peripheral neuropathy. *Neu-
    rology* 1992;42:14–18.
Dyck PJ, Dyck JB, Grant IA, et al. Ten steps in characterizing and diag-
    nosing patients with peripheral neuropathy. *Neurology* 1996;47:
    10–17.
Poncelet AN. An algorithm for the evaluation of peripheral neuropathy.
    Am Fam Physician 1998;57:755–764.
Ropper AH. The Guillain-Barre syndrome. *N Engl J Med* 1992;326:
    1130–1136.

Chapter 9

Spinal Cord Compression

Case

A 64-year-old woman with known multiple myeloma has a 1-week history of sharp back pain radiating around the left costal margin that is worse with coughing. For the past day she has noticed incontinence of urine, and during the past 5 hours she has become weak in her legs. Decadron is given intravenously, and emergency magnetic resonance imaging (MRI) of the spine shows an epidural mass at T6, with cord compression. She is started treatment with radiation therapy that night, and during a 2-week period gradually improves to her baseline.

Diagnosis

Acute spinal cord compression, T6, caused by epidural bony metastasis from multiple myeloma.

Acute spinal cord compression is a neurologic emergency. Prognosis is related to the delay between onset of neurologic symptoms and treatment. Being alert to the possibility of cord compression is crucial for early diagnosis.

CHARACTERISTIC SYMPTOMS

1. Back pain
2. Root pain, often radiating around the side or down a limb
3. Paresthesias in legs ("funny feelings," tingling, or numbness)

4. Change in urine function (patient urinates more or less frequently or is incontinent)
5. Weakness in lower extremities (especially when climbing stairs)
6. Constipation or fecal incontinence

EARLY SIGNS

1. Loss of pinprick sensation or a different reaction to pinprick in the lower extremities. The patient may have a sensory "level" to pinprick. There may be a temperature "level" to a cool object or a "sweat" level.
2. Altered position or vibration sensation below the level of the lesion.
3. Tenderness over the spine is a helpful sign in determining the level of the lesion.
4. Hyperreflexia below the level of the lesion. If the lesion is in the thoracic cord, legs are hyperreflexic compared with arms.
5. Signs are usually bilateral (i.e., both legs, both arms) rather than unilateral.

Note: The toes are often down-going, and reflexes may be reduced in early acute cord compression because of spinal shock.

LATE SIGNS

1. Definite weakness
2. Definite hyperreflexia
3. Up-going toes
4. A sensory level to pinprick, temperature, or vibration; it is often helpful to check vibration sense up and down the spine in search of a level; check for a sweat level
5. Loss of anal sphincter tone and voluntary contraction; absent abdominal reflexes; absent bulbocavernosus reflex
6. Urinary retention or incontinence of bowel or bladder

CAUSES OF SPINAL CORD COMPRESSION

Epidural Compression

1. Metastatic tumor (especially from lung, breast, and prostate); spinal cord compression may be the initial manifestation of malignancy

2. Trauma
3. Lymphoma
4. Multiple myeloma
5. Epidural abscess or hematoma
6. Cervical or thoracic disc protrusion or spondylosis or spondylolisthesis
7. Atlantoaxial subluxation (rheumatoid arthritis)

Extramedullary, Intradural Compression

1. Meningioma
2. Neurofibroma

Intramedullary Expansion

1. Glioma
2. Ependymoma
3. Arteriovenous malformation

DIAGNOSTIC STEPS

1. Perform a careful neurologic examination; estimate the level of the cord lesion. Note that the lesion may lie above the sensory level because of partial injury and lamination of sensory tracts. Also note that the dermatomal level does not correspond to the bony level because of the termination of the cord at about T12-L1 (Fig. 9.1).
2. Check for primary tumor sites (e.g., careful examination of breast, nodes, and prostate; chest radiograph; routine laboratory studies, including complete blood count, liver function test, and prostate specific antigen).
3. Plain films of the spine may reveal (a) vertebral collapse or subluxation, (b) bony erosion secondary to tumor, or (c) calcification (meningioma).
4. Early consultation with a neurologist or neurosurgeon and a radiation therapist is needed.
5. Perform an MRI scan of the spine with sagittal cuts through the entire spine and axial cuts through suspicious areas. If the patient cannot tolerate an MRI, a computed tomographic myelogram usually is done. MRI has become the diagnostic study of choice in acute cord compression. If myelography is necessary and if a spinal block is seen on

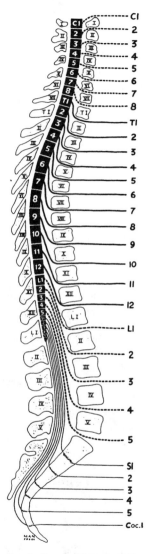

FIGURE 9.1. (Reproduced with permission from Haymaker W, Woodhall B. *Peripheral nerve injuries.* Philadelphia: WB Saunders, 1945.)

myelogram, image above the block using a cisternal puncture to examine the extent of disease.

6. Do not perform a lumbar puncture if cord compression is suspected; imaging the lesion is the initial key to diagnosis and treatment.

7. Image the entire spine if possible. There may be multiple sites of compression, which influences therapy.

TREATMENT

Treatment depends on the site(s) of cord injury and the etiology. Treatment is most effective if instituted early. Acute bowel and bladder dysfunction in the setting of cord compression is an emergency, as is rapidly progressive weakness. Modalities include radiotherapy (for such disorders as metastatic breast or prostate cancer or Hodgkin's lymphoma), surgical decompression for solitary radioresistant extradural solid tumors, or a combination of both. Dexamethasone (16 to 60 mg intravenously) usually is given immediately when compression is suspected clinically because it may help to preserve spinal cord function. A dose of dexamethasone should be continued into radiotherapy and then tapered. A specific protocol for traumatic spinal cord injury may improve functional outcome (see Suggested Reading).

DIFFERENTIAL DIAGNOSIS OF NONCOMPRESSIVE SPINAL CORD INJURY

1. *Transverse myelitis* is characterized by the acute or subacute development of paraplegia or quadriplegia, occasionally asymmetric, associated with back pain and sensory loss. It may be related to a preceding viral illness (e.g., mononucleosis). The cerebrospinal fluid may show pleocytosis with increased protein and normal sugar levels. Studies for disorders such as Lyme disease, lupus erythematosus, syphilis, human immunodeficiency virus, cytomegalovirus, and herpes simplex virus should be considered. Myelography or MRI is usually necessary to rule out a compressive lesion. In addition, MRI may show intramedullary pathology such as a plaque of demyelinating disease. Treatment is supportive. Corticosteroids often are used when the etiology is thought to be postinfectious or demyelinating.

2. *Radiation myelopathy* usually occurs 6 months to 5 years after irradiation to the thoracic area of the spinal cord (e.g., for lymphoma). Onset may be insidious or abrupt and may be limited to paresthesias or progress to actual paralysis. MRI or myelography is needed to rule out a compressive lesion and may show intrinsic cord abnormalities. There is no known treatment, and the myelopathy is probably secondary to vascular damage to the spinal cord. Steroids or anticoagulants have been tried in such cases.

3. *Acute myelopathy* also may be secondary to toxins (e.g., heroin, arsenic), associated with malignancy elsewhere in the body as a remote effect, or secondary to vascular infarction of the spinal cord caused by anterior spinal artery occlusion. In the latter condition, motor function and pain and temperature appreciation are affected, whereas position and vibration sense (posterior column functions) are spared.

4. Acute spinal cord trauma is treated with stabilization of the spine and with methylprednisolone according to a specific infusion protocol depending on the time after injury.

Suggested Reading

Bracken MB, Shepard MJ, Holford TR, et al. Administration of methyl-prednisolone for 24 or 48 hours or Trilazad Mesylate for 48 hours in the treatment of acute spinal cord injury. *JAMA* 1997;277: 1597–1604.

Byrne TN. Spinal cord compression from epidural metastases. *N Engl J Med* 1992;327:614–619.

Chiles BW, Cooper PR. Acute spinal injury. *N Engl J Med* 1996;334: 514–520.

Dawson DM, Potts F. Acute nontraumatic myelopathies. *Neurol Clin* 1991; 9;585–603.

Ditunno JF, Formal CS. Chronic spinal cord injury. *N Engl J Med* 1994; 330:550–556.

Grant R, Papadopoulos SM, Greenberg HS. Metastatic epidural spinal cord compression. *Neurol Clin* 1991;9:825–842.

Rowland LP. Surgical treatment of cervical spondylotic myelopathy: time for a controlled trial. *Neurology* 1992;42:5–13.

Wagner R, Jagoda A. Spinal cord syndromes. *Emerg Med Clin North Am* 1997;15:699–711.

Chapter 10

Peripheral Nerve and Root Dysfunction

Case

A 27-year-old avid cyclist competes in road races. She uses a pair of cycling gloves, but in long distance races has a habit of staying in the "drops," with her hand clenched firmly at the base of the handlebars. That forces the medial side of her wrist up against the bar. After a double century ride (200 miles), she notices pain over the pisiform bone and weakness of abduction and adduction of the fingers. She has no numbness but has some twitching of the first dorsal interosseus muscle. After 6 weeks, her symptoms resolve spontaneously.

Diagnosis

Pressure induced mononeuropathy, ulnar nerve, at the wrist.

To diagnose peripheral nerve and root injuries, one must determine which muscles are affected, outline the territory of sensory loss, and note any reflex changes. One then compares this distribution with the known territories supplied by nerves or roots to localize the lesion.

Reflexes

Reflexes are diminished in root and peripheral nerve disease. Root irritation alone or damage to a root not involved in the reflex arc does not decrease the reflex. There are four primary reflexes to remember, with particular roots and muscles necessary for their function. An easy way to learn the roots is to remember that, going from ankle to triceps, the roots are numbered consecutively from one to eight (Table 10.1).

TABLE 10.1.   Four Primary Reflexes

Reflex	Roots Needed for Reflex	Muscle Carrying Out the Reflex
Ankle jerk	S1	Gastrocnemius
Knee jerk	L2, L3, L4	Quadriceps
Biceps	C5, C6	Biceps
Triceps	C7, C8	Triceps

ROOTS AND MUSCLES

Each muscle is supplied by two or more roots. Thus, weakness associated with injury to only one root is partial, as opposed to peripheral nerve injury, which may cause complete muscle weakness. Nevertheless, certain muscles tend to be preferentially supplied by certain roots, so that they are particularly affected by injury to the root. Table 10.2 describes the most useful muscles

TABLE 10.2.   Roots and the Primary Muscles They Supply

Route	Muscle	Action
C5	Deltoid	Shoulder abduction
C5	Infraspinatus	Humeral external rotation (Check: have patient externally rotate the humerus with the arm held at side and flexed at the elbow, as if shooting a gun)
C5, C6	Biceps	Flexion of the supinated forearm
C6	Extensor carpi radialis and ulnaris	Wrist extension
C7	Extensors digitorum	Finger extensions; forearm extension at elbow
	Triceps	
C8, T1	Interossei and lumbricals	Digital abduction and adduction (Check: have patient move fingers apart and together against resistance)
L2, L3, L4	Quadriceps, iliopsoas	Knee extension, thigh on hip flexion
	Adductor group	Thigh adduction
L5	Anterior tibial and extensor hallucis	Ankle and large toe dorsiflexion (Check: have patient walk on heels)
S1	Gastrocnemius	Ankle plantar flexion (Check: have patient walk on tiptoes)

to test for root injury and which roots supply each muscle. Each root has a sensory distribution as represented on the standard dermatome chart (see Chapter 34). The most useful root dermatomes to remember are C2 over the posterior head, C4 the shoulder, C7 the middle finger, T4 the nipple, T10 the umbilicus, L3 the knee, S1 the lateral foot, and S3,4,5 the anal region.

NERVES AND MUSCLES OF THE UPPER EXTREMITY

Median Nerve

The median nerve (C6-T1) originates in the brachial plexus and supplies two basic muscle groups:

1. *Forearm*: pronator of the forearm, radial flexion, and wrist abduction
2. *Hand*: the first two *L*umbricales (index and middle finger flexion at the metacarpophalangeal joint), thumb *O*pposition with opponens pollicis, *A*bduction with abductor pollicis brevis, and *F*lexion with flexor pollicis brevis ("LOAF" muscles)

Sensory loss involves the thumb, index, and middle fingers and half of the ring finger (Fig. 10.1).

Clinical comment: A complete median nerve lesion (forearm and hand muscles) is usually secondary to traumatic injury in the

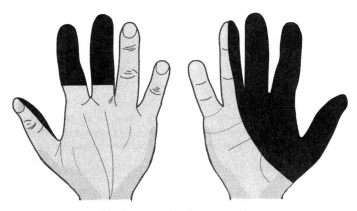

FIGURE 10.1. Median sensory loss.

axilla or to a lesion affecting the median nerve at the elbow. Entrapment of the anterior interosseus branch causes weakness of thumb distal flexion and flexion of the distal phalanx of the second and third digits. Entrapment at the wrist is common after wrist fractures. A clinical syndrome of median entrapment at the wrist with intermittent or progressive symptoms is called the "carpal tunnel syndrome." Patients with this syndrome often complain of numbness and tingling in the thumb and first two fingers; the hands typically "fall asleep" with use or at night (nocturnal paresthesias). The earliest weakness is a difficulty twisting jar lids open or a tendency to drop objects. Muscle wasting and obvious loss of power occurs later. The diagnosis may be confirmed by nerve conduction studies. The carpal tunnel syndrome is often bilateral and may be associated with systemic processes; consider rheumatoid arthritis, hypothyroidism, diabetes, pregnancy, gout, acromegaly, and amyloidosis. Medical management includes treating the underlying disease, splinting the wrist, and injecting steroids into the carpal tunnel. Surgical decompression of the carpal tunnel may be necessary and is usually successful.

Ulnar Nerve

The ulnar nerve (C8-T1) supplies muscles and sensory areas on the palm not supplied by the median nerve. When ulnar nerve disease is suspected, think of little finger and hypothenar eminence. The ulnar nerve runs in the ulnar groove at the medial aspect of the elbow ("funny bone") and supplies the following two muscle groups:

1. *Forearm*: ulnar flexion at the wrist
2. *Hand*: little finger abduction and opposition, thumb adduction, all the interosseous muscles (used to spread fingers apart and bring together), third and fourth lumbricales (ring and little finger flexion at the metacarpophalangeal joint)

Sensory loss involves half of the fourth finger and the little finger (Fig. 10.2).

Clinical comment: The ulnar nerve commonly is injured at the elbow, where it is most exposed. Tardive (delayed) ulnar palsy may occur years after trauma to the elbow (perhaps when fibrosis becomes significant). Look for muscle weakness as opposed to

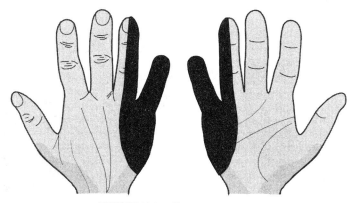

FIGURE 10.2. Ulnar sensory loss.

the prominent sensory symptoms seen in median nerve dysfunction. A claw hand, caused by trauma, surgery, or tumor at the apex of the lung, also is seen with involvement of C8-T1 roots at the origin of the brachial plexus: check for Homer's syndrome (small pupil and ptosis) on the same side as the claw hand. This indicates sympathetic fiber involvement in the area of the brachial plexus. C8-T1 and lower trunk lesions involve distal muscles of the median and radial nerve, such as the extensor of the forefinger (radial nerve) and the abductor pollicis brevis (median nerve).

Radial Nerve

The radial nerve (C5-C8) winds around the humerus in the spiral groove, then travels in the lateral aspect of the elbow. When there is a wrist drop, think of radial nerve injury.

The radial nerve supplies these muscles:

1. *Supinator* of the forearm; the brachioradialis reflex may be lost.
2. *Extensors* of the fingers, wrist, elbow (triceps), and thumb.

Sensory loss involves the back of the hand and is not always present (Fig. 10.3).

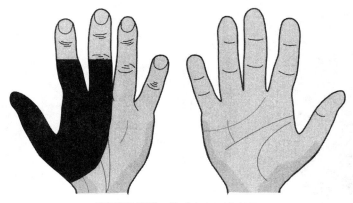

FIGURE 10.3. Radial sensory loss.

Clinical comment: Injury to the radial nerve may occur in the axilla (e.g., after using crutches), giving inability to extend the elbow, and may include wrist drop. If the radial nerve is involved at the humerus, only wrist drop is found. Pressure palsies are common ("Bridegroom's palsy," when the groom sleeps with the bride's head on his arm). In addition, the radial nerve is affected in diabetes and lead poisoning. In radial nerve palsy, the ability to spread the fingers apart (ulnar nerve function) may be weak because of the mechanical disadvantage caused by the wrist drop. Check with wrist resting on a flat surface (e.g., table) to overcome that handicap.

Thoracic Outlet Syndrome

The thoracic outlet syndrome refers to symptoms and signs that occur because of compression of the subclavian vessels and brachial plexus at the superior aperture of the thorax between the first rib and the clavicle. Previously thought to be common, it is now clear that true neurogenic or vascular thoracic outlet syndrome is rare. Symptoms include pain and paresthesias in the neck, shoulder, arm, and hand (C8, Tl distribution); weakness of the hand; change of color of the hand, including pallor of the fingers; and aggravation of all symptoms by use of the upper limb. Signs depend on whether primarily vascular or neural compression exists and include supraclavicular bruit, loss or diminution of radial pulse, weakness and sensory loss in the hand, and reproduction of pain by pressure in the supraclavicular fossa or by traction on the arm. Anomalies of the spine often are present, including cervical ribs or abnormal transverse process of C7. More commonly, pain in the shoulder or pain in the arm is attributed to thoracic outlet syndrome without good supportive data. The diagnosis of thoracic outlet syndrome should be made only when definite nerve conduction or electromyogram data support the neurogenic form or when there is evidence of vascular disease supporting the vascular form.

Cervical Radiculopathy

"Radiculopathy" refers to a disorder of an individual nerve root. A herniated disc causing nerve root compression should be suspected when there is neck pain; pain shooting down the arm ("radicular pain"); and evidence of sensory, motor, and reflex change conforming to the distribution of one or more cervical roots. Root lesions give prominent pain and sensory loss with milder weakness. This is because each muscle is supplied by two or more nerve roots, so with individual root lesions, weakness is incomplete (see Table 10.2).

Cervical Spondylosis

"Spondylosis" refers to degenerative aging changes of the spine. Osteophyte formation, disk degeneration, and hypertrophic changes in ligaments all are part of this process. Check for (a) multiple, often asymmetric, root involvement in the upper extremities, with muscle wasting and hypoactive reflexes in the distribution of those roots affected and (b) compression of the cervical spinal cord, giving hyperactive lower-extremity reflexes, up-going toes, and leg weakness. Remember, sensory symptoms in the hands plus spastic lower extremities in patients older than age 50 years equal cervical spondylosis with myelopathy until proved otherwise. Similar symptoms may be caused by foramen magnum tumors or anomalies of the posterior fossa such as Chiari malformations, especially in younger patients.

NERVES AND MUSCLES OF THE LOWER EXTREMITY

Obturator Nerve

The obturator nerve (L2-L3-L4 roots, ventral portion) supplies the adductors of the thigh (brings legs together). It may be damaged during labor, involved in diabetes, or affected by local pelvic disease or by obturator hernia (Table 10.3).

Femoral Nerve

The femoral nerve (L2-L3-L4 roots, dorsal portion) supplies the iliopsoas (hip flexion) and quadriceps (knee extension). The knee jerk is diminished or absent. Numbness extends over the thigh and down the medial shin. Femoral nerve involvement may be distinguished from root involvement at L2-L3-L4 (e.g., by paravertebral tumor) by checking thigh adduction (obturator), which is affected if roots are involved but spared if only the femoral nerve is involved. Causes of femoral neuropathy include diabetes (look for quadriceps wasting with pain over the anterior thigh), tumor, polyarteritis, pelvic trauma, and hemorrhage into the iliacus muscle in patients taking anticoagulants.

Lateral Femoral Cutaneous Nerve

The lateral femoral cutaneous nerve is a pure sensory nerve (L2-L3) that supplies the lateral thigh. Injury to this nerve causes tingling, burning, and pain, which is often worse with standing. The lateral femoral cutaneous nerve syndrome ("meralgia paraesthetica") is common in diabetes and may appear during pregnancy or as a result of pressure from a tight-fitting belt, obesity, or even poor posture. Treatment involves removing the offend-

TABLE 10.3. Characteristic Features Associated with Various Nerves

Nerve	Involvement
Median	Thumb and thenar eminence
Ulnar	Little finger and hypothenar eminence
Radial	Wrist-drop
Femoral	Absent knee jerk, weak hip flexion and knee extension
Peroneal	Foot-drop
Sciatic	Pain down lateral thigh and leg, often with absent ankle jerk

ing agent, and, if necessary, injecting the nerve with steroids at its entrance to the thigh or surgical release. Meralgia paresthetica is a common cause of referral to neurologists. A loose belt, weight loss, and nonsteroidal medications are often effective treatment strategies.

Sciatic Nerve

The sciatic nerve (L4-S3) supplies hamstrings (flexion of the knee) and all muscles below the knee. At the knee, it divides into the *peroneal nerve*, which runs anteriorly and supplies muscles that dorsiflex and evert the foot and provide sensation on top of the foot, and the *tibial nerve*, which runs posteriorly at the knee and supplies muscles of plantar flexion and inversion and sensation on the sole of the foot.

Clinically, the most common affliction of the sciatic nerve is "sciatica," a syndrome of pain radiating down the leg from the buttock or back. Irritation of any root from L4-S3 may produce sciatica to a varying degree. One of the most common causes of sciatica is lumbar disc protrusion (pain may be precipitated by coughing or sneezing), often with associated reflex loss and weakness in a root distribution. Straight leg raising generally aggravates the pain. Some patients may have no neurologic findings with a herniated disc, although often there is paravertebral muscle spasm. If root dysfunction occurs, this may help localize the disc protrusion level (Table 10.4). However, far lateral or far medial disc protrusions may affect the roots above or below the "usual" level, respectively (Fig. 10.4).

Treatment
Because low back pain and sciatica are frequently benign and transient, a conservative course of treatment within the first few

TABLE 10.4.   Most Common Lumbar Disc Syndromes

Root	Disc Interspace	Reflex Affected	Motor Weakness	Sensory Changes (If Any)
L4	L3-L4	Knee jerk	Knee extension	Anterior thigh
L5	L4-L5	Hamstring jerk	Great toe dorsiflexion	Great toe
S1	L5-S1	Ankle jerk	Foot, plantar flexion	Foot, lateral border

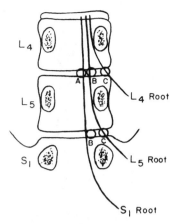

FIGURE 10.4. Disc protrusions. **A.** Very medial disc protrusion. **B.** Posterolateral disc protrusion. **C.** Very lateral disc protrusion. (From Brazis P, Masdeu JC, Biller J. *Localization in clinical neurology*, 2nd ed. Boston: Little, Brown & Company, 1996, with permission.)

weeks is recommended, unless there is evidence to suggest more severe neurologic dysfunction or an unusual cause of sciatica. Bed rest for 3 days is as effective as more prolonged bed rest, and the use of pain medications or nonsteroidal medications may help in pain relief. A course of physiotherapy may be helpful. Epidural steroids have been shown to have only a transient effect in relieving pain from disc protrusion and do not provide a long-term functional benefit or reduce the ultimate need for surgical treatment. If conservative management is unsuccessful or if there is significant neurologic dysfunction, magnetic resonance imaging (MRI) or computed tomography (CT) scanning of the lumbar spine is usually effective in defining the pathology. If necessary, myelography with follow-up CT may show far lateral disc protrusions not visible on MRI. Surgical decompression of discs usually is considered when medical management fails.

Peroneal Nerve

The peroneal nerve supplies dorsiflexors (tibialis anterior) and everters (turning out) of the foot. Inverters (turning in) of the foot are supplied by the tibial nerve. The sensory distribution involves the lateral aspect of the leg and dorsum of the foot.

Clinically, peroneal nerve palsy gives foot drop and is analogous to wrist drop (radial nerve) in the upper extremity. Foot drop is seen in diabetes and is a frequent pressure palsy from trauma or pressure in a thin or wasted individual because of the superficial location of the nerve at the head of the fibula by the knee. Hereditary peroneal neuropathy (Charcot-Marie-Tooth disease) is associated with bilateral foot drop, a wasted anterior leg compartment below the knee, and pes cavus. Remember, peroneal palsy spares the inverters of the foot; if the inverters are also weak, the lesion is higher, generally at the sciatic nerve, root, or cord level. Although peroneal palsy is the most common cause of foot drop, the differential diagnosis of foot drop includes the following:

1. Sciatic nerve injury. *Clue*: Tibialis posterior is affected, as are other muscles supplied by sciatic nerve, such as gastrocnemius.
2. L5 nerve root. *Clue*: Tibialis posterior is affected, often with associated back pain.
3. Spinal cord. *Clue*: Upper motor neuron signs (e.g., Babinski) are present.
4. Hemisphere. *Clue*: Anterior cerebral infarct causes other signs of hemiparesis and frontal lobe signs.

Posterior Tibial Nerve

The posterior tibial nerve rarely is injured alone because it runs deep in the calf. It may be entrapped distally in the tarsal tunnel, causing pain in the sole of the foot.

CONUS MEDULLARIS AND CAUDA EQUINA LESIONS

The conus medullaris (lower sacral segments of the spinal cord) and cauda equina (elongated roots of the lumbar and sacral spinal nerves) can be affected by a variety of processes. Differential diagnosis includes tumor, hemorrhage, disc herniation, pelvic fracture, spondylolisthesis, and inflammatory lesions. Helpful distinguishing features are contained in Table 10.5. In either case, neurosurgical evaluation is warranted.

TABLE 10.5.   Distinguishing Features of Conus Medullaris and Cauda Equina Lesions

	Conus Medullaris	Cauda Equina
Motor weakness	Absent or mild	Present and usually unilateral
Sensory deficits	Bilateral (saddle)	Usually unilateral
Sphincter involvement	Early; of bladder and bowel	Late and mild

INVESTIGATION OF NERVE AND ROOT DYSFUNCTION

Examine the patient to determine whether the nerve or root is involved. Determine whether the sensory loss (or symptom) and muscle weakness (if present) fit the distribution of a particular nerve or root.

Establish the Etiology

1. Did a nerve palsy come on after *sleep or surgery* (pressure palsies)?
2. Is there evidence of *trauma*? If so, is it old or new?
3. What are the patient's *occupation* and habits? For example, there may be median nerve involvement in computer users and beauty operators or ulnar nerve damage in cyclists.
4. Is there evidence of *systemic disease* (e.g., diabetes, uremia, breast cancer affecting the brachial plexus, polyarteritis, granulomatous infection, human immunodeficiency virus infection, nutritional deficiency)?

CRANIAL NERVE DISORDERS

The cranial nerves are complex, and an extensive discussion of their functions and courses is best seen in texts of neuroanatomy. The most useful cranial nerves to test in a clinical setting include the following:

- II: optic nerve, visual fields
- III, IV, VI: pupil, eye movements
- V: facial sensation, jaw movement
- VII: facial movement, tearing, salivation
- VIII: hearing, balance
- IX, X: gag and swallowing
- XII: tongue movement

Trigeminal Neuralgia

Excruciating, paroxysmal pain lasting seconds to minutes in the distribution of the second or third division of the fifth cranial nerve is the hallmark of trigeminal neuralgia (tic douloureux). The pain often is "triggered" by touching the side of the face or is brought on by facial movement, such as chewing. There is no objective motor or sensory loss. The cause is unknown but may be related to a viral infection or to pressure on the nerve by a small vessel in the root entry zone. Trigeminal neuralgia is uncommon in people younger than age 40 years. When it occurs in the young patient, particularly if associated with objective sensory loss, it is frequently secondary to multiple sclerosis. Neurologic signs (loss of sensation on the face, cranial nerve palsies, long tract signs) suggest focal pathology, such as tumor, vascular malformation, or demyelinating disease. Approximately 10% of patients with trigeminal neuralgia have a structural lesion. Treatment with carbamazepine relieves pain in most patients (begin with 100 mg twice a day; increase by 100 mg/day up to 1,200 mg/day; monitor hematologic indices). Other drugs, such as phenytoin, baclofen, gabapentin, and lamotrigine may be useful. Trigeminal neuralgia refractory to medical treatment may require surgical intervention. Glycerol injection or balloon ablation of the nerve may be effective. Percutaneous radiofrequency coagulation of the gasserian ganglion may be effective in relieving the pain of trigeminal neuralgia. Some patients may require vascular decompression of the trigeminal nerve via craniotomy. The latter procedure carries a 1% mortality, which limits its use.

Seventh Nerve Palsies

Peripheral involvement of the seventh cranial nerve is a well-recognized syndrome. Onset may be heralded by pain behind the ear, and diagnosis is based on demonstrating complete facial palsy (i.e., paralysis of both lower face and forehead) in the absence of other neurologic findings. Central lesions that affect fibers before their synapse in the seventh nerve nucleus in the brainstem spare forehead musculature. In addition to innervating facial musculature, fibers from the seventh nerve innervate the lacrimal gland of the eye (decreasing tearing), the stapedius muscle in the ear (hyperacusis), and the submaxillary and sublingual glands, and they carry afferent taste fibers from the ante-

rior two thirds of the tongue (loss of taste). Most cases are idiopathic (Bell's palsy). Other causes include infectious mononucleosis, Lyme disease, the Guillain-Barré syndrome (bilateral seventh nerve palsies, loss of reflexes), fracture, severe
hypertension, diabetes, sarcoid and histiocytosis, and an associated otitis or mastoiditis. Herpes zoster may affect the seventh
nerve, causing facial palsy and cutaneous vesicles in the external
ear (Ramsay Hunt syndrome). A cerebellopontine angle tumor
or a brainstem plaque from multiple sclerosis may give a peripheral seventh nerve palsy, usually in association with other cranial
nerve signs. Melkersson's syndrome is recurrent seventh nerve
palsies associated with facial edema.

Treatment

Treatment with prednisone probably hastens recovery and the
amount of residual facial disfiguration in the idiopathic variety
(Bell's palsy) and should be administered within the first 72
hours of onset (60 mg/day for 4 days, then taper over 10 days).
Acyclovir therapy in combination with steroid therapy is more
effective than steroid therapy alone. An eye shield and methyl-
cellulose eye drops will help prevent corneal ulceration, but
patching the eye may cause irritation. Surgical decompression of
the facial nerve is probably of no benefit. Recovery usually begins
within 1 to 4 weeks of onset and may take longer than 3 months
to be complete. Patients with hyperacusis, taste loss, or defective
tearing have a poorer prognosis (proximal lesion of the facial
nerve), as do those with complete (as opposed to partial) facial
nerve paralysis. Search specifically for involvement of sixth and
fifth cranial nerves, which lie close to the seventh nerve in the
brainstem and in the peripheral course of the nerve.

Suggested Reading

Aids to the investigation of peripheral nerve injuries. London: Her Majesty's
    Stationery Office, 1986.
Anto C, Aradhya P. Clinical diagnosis of peripheral nerve compression in
    the upper extremity. *Orthop Clin North Am* 1996;27:227–236.
Carette S, Marcoux S, Truchon R, et al. A controlled trial of corticoster-
    oid injections into facet joints for chronic low back pain. *N Engl J
    Med* 1991;325:1002–1007.
Dawson D. Entrapment neuropathies of the upper extremities. *N Engl J
    Med* 1993;329:2013–2018.

Dellon AL, Hament W, Gittelshon A. Nonoperative management of cubital tunnel syndrome: an 8-year prospective study. *Neurology* 1993; 43:1673–1677.

Feinberg JH, Nadler SF, Krivickas LS. Peripheral nerve injuries in the athlete. *Sports Med* 1997;24:385–408.

Morgenlander JC, Lynch JR, Sanders DB. Surgical treatment of carpal tunnel syndrome in patients with peripheral neuropathy. *Neurology* 1997;49:1159–1163.

Nakano KK. Nerve entrapment syndromes. *Curr Opin Rheumatol* 1997;9: 165–173.

Report of the quality standards subcommittee of the American Academy of Neurology. Practice parameters for carpal tunnel syndrome. *Neurology* 1993;43:2406–2409.

Sunderland S. *Nerves and nerve injuries*. London: Churchill Livingstone, 1978.

Von Korff M, Barlow W, Cherkin D, et al. Effects of practice style in managing back pain. *Ann Intern Med* 1994;121:187–195.

Chapter 11

Muscle Weakness

Case

A 43-year-old man has a 6-week history of difficulty getting out of bed, arising from a chair, combing his hair, and going up stairs. He has noticed an unusual rash on his knuckles and around his eyelids. He has lost some weight and feels generally fatigued. His medical health has otherwise been normal, and he ingests no toxins and is a nonsmoker and nondrinker. His examination shows proximal muscle weakness, normal deep tendon reflexes and sensory examination, down-going toes, and a rash on his hands and face. His creatine kinase is 805 units, four times the upper limit of normal.

Diagnosis

Dermatomyositis

When confronted with a patient who has muscle weakness (Table 11.1), the physician must establish whether the weakness is myopathic; whether the myopathy is congenital or acquired; and if acquired, whether it represents a manifestation of another illness (e.g., thyroid myopathy). Patients with neuromuscular junction disorders have proximal muscle weakness that is fatigable, as well as ocular, facial, and gustatory muscle weakness.

HISTORY

In patients with muscle weakness caused by a myopathy, the following occurs:

TABLE 11.1. Myopathies and Related Disorders

Acquired myopathies

Polymyositis (idiopathic or associated with tumor)

Endocrinopathies

Steroid-associated

Alcoholic

Metabolic

Inclusion body myositis

Muscular dystrophies (onset after age 30 is rare)

Duchenne: affects young boys, death by age 20

Facioscapulohumeral: autosomal dominant, onset from ages 10 to 20

Limb-girdle: affects shoulder and pelvis musculature, onset from ages 15 to 25

Myotonic dystrophy: usually manifests in early adult life with myotonia, peripheral muscle wasting, endocrinopathies, impotence, frontal balding, cataracts; inheritance is autosomal dominant

Neuromuscular junction disorders

Myasthenia gravis: classically involves ocular muscles, and variability is characteristic; there may be proximal muscle weakness although myasthenia gravis is not a myopathy

Lambert-Eaton syndrome: usually seen with underlying carcinoma of the lung

1. Weakness comes on gradually rather than suddenly.
2. Weakness is usually symmetric and proximal, with the shoulder and pelvic girdle muscles most severely affected. Climbing stairs, squatting, arising from a chair, and combing the hair are particularly difficult.
3. There are no sensory symptoms (i.e., no "pins-and-needles" sensations or loss of sensation), which are common in neuropathies.
4. Bowel and bladder function are spared.
5. Weakness is usually painless.
6. Cramps may be present, but spasticity is not a feature of the weakness. Spasticity suggests an upper motor neuron problem.

In patients with neuromuscular junction disorders, the following occurs:

1. Weakness tends to be fluctuating and worse after exercise or later in the day.

2. Weakness is symmetric and proximal.
3. There may be diplopia, facial muscle weakness, and neck weakness.
4. Swallowing and respiration may be affected.

Establish the following points:

1. Is there a *family history* of similar disorders? Muscular dystrophies are often familial.
2. Is there *myotonia* (unable to release grip, slowness to initiate muscle movements)?
3. Is there *trouble swallowing*? This is seen frequently in polymyositis.
4. Is there a variation during the day, *fatigability*, or diplopia? This is suggestive of neuromuscular junction disorders such as myasthenia gravis.
5. What was the exact *age of onset*? This may help distinguish congenital from acquired myopathies.

PHYSICAL EXAMINATION

In the patient with myopathy:

1. *Proximal limb strength* is more impaired than distal strength except in certain muscular dystrophies. Check deltoids (shoulder), neck flexion, and iliopsoas (hip flexion). Check neck flexion (which is weaker than neck extension). Weakness tends to be distal in neuropathies, and there are usually sensory symptoms and a loss of reflexes. Weakness may be proximal in Guillain-Barré syndrome, but there are areflexia, sensory symptoms, and increased cerebrospinal fluid (CSF) protein levels.
2. *Reflexes* are preserved or slightly decreased except in later stages of muscle weakness.
3. *Sensation* is normal.

Check these points, which help to distinguish one cause of muscle weakness from another:

1. Certain muscular dystrophies have a typical pattern. Check for *facial muscle involvement* in fascioscapulohumeral dystrophy. Have the patient shut eyes tightly, puff cheeks, or attempt to whistle (difficult in fascioscapulohumeral). See if

pelvic and thigh muscles are most involved, possibly indicating a limb-girdle dystrophy. Check for *myotonia* by percussing the muscles directly, tapping the tongue, and having the patient close the eyes tightly to see if the patient has trouble opening them. Patients with myotonia may have trouble "letting go" in a handshake. Such signs are seen in myotonia congenita, myotonic dystrophy, and other myotonic disorders.

2. Check for fatigability and involvement of extraocular muscles, particularly when facial weakness occurs with eyelid ptosis. These are suggestive of neuromuscular junction disorders. Many patients with myasthenia gravis also have dysphagia and dysarthria and may resort to holding the jaw closed as they eat.

LABORATORY STUDIES

Characteristic features of myopathies include the following:

1. Elevated muscle enzymes, especially creatine phosphokinase (CPK) and aldolase.
2. Normal spinal fluid, including CSF protein.

Special studies usually conducted on patients suspected of having myopathies are as follows:

1. *Electromyography (EMG) and nerve conduction studies.* EMG should demonstrate small, polyphasic, early recruiting motor units in the involved muscles consistent with myopathy. Polymyositis may show "irritative features" with fibrillation potentials and high-frequency repetitive discharges. Nerve conduction studies are usually normal.
2. *Muscle biopsy.* Make sure to conduct a biopsy on an affected muscle, and avoid biopsy of a muscle previously used for EMG to avoid artifact from needle insertion.

IS THERE A TREATABLE MUSCLE WEAKNESS PRESENT?

Check for the following:

1. *Thyroid myopathy.* Myopathy may occur with hyperthyroidism or hypothyroidism. Periodic paralysis is a feature in some patients with Graves' disease.

2. *Steroid myopathy.* This commonly occurs in patients taking steroids for other conditions, as well as in Cushing's disease. Steroids may exacerbate the myopathy seen in critically ill patients in the intensive care unit (ICU). The CPK is usually normal.

3. *Statin-associated myositis.* Patients taking cholesterol-lowering agents may develop a painful myositis, which improves when the statin is withdrawn.

4. *Polymyositis.* There is usually an elevated sedimentation rate and, at times, evidence of other connective tissue disease, such as rheumatoid arthritis or lupus erythematosus. Skin changes with characteristic heliotrope rash are seen with dermatomyositis. Treatment of idiopathic polymyositis includes steroids and immunosuppressant therapy. Approximately 20% of adults with polymyositis have an underlying malignancy.

   Note: *Inclusion body myositis may be confused with polymyositis.* Most patients are middle-aged or elderly men with slowly progressive symmetric weakness. Women are less commonly affected and more likely to be younger. In contrast to other inflammatory myopathies, distal weakness is often as severe as proximal weakness and may include weakness of foot extensors and finger flexors. Pain is uncommon. Most patients have a protracted course that is generally unaffected by the usual immunosuppressive therapies. Muscle biopsy shows typical "inclusion bodies."

5. *Alcoholic myopathy.* These patients may have a subacute and sometimes painful myopathy associated with excessive alcohol ingestion. Does the patient have a concurrent alcoholic cardiac myopathy or neuropathy? Make sure to inquire about alcohol consumption.

6. *Periodic paralysis.* Patients usually have a family history and describe attacks of diffuse muscle weakness lasting hours. Attacks are provoked by cold, food, or exercise, and patients may have a variety of inherited muscle membrane disorders, sometimes characterized by the abnormal potassium level at the time of the attack. Myotonia may be present in the hyperkalemic form.

7. *Polymyalgia rheumatica.* This usually occurs in elderly patients with muscle aches in the shoulder girdle and hip girdle. Sed-

imentation rate is elevated, and the disorder responds to low-dose steroids. Some of these patients harbor concurrent temporal arteritis.

8. *Myasthenia gravis.* The etiology of myasthenia is an autoimmune attack on acetylcholine receptors of the postsynaptic part of the neuromuscular junction. The patients usually have fluctuating weakness—worse later in the day—often with ptosis, diplopia, and difficulty swallowing. The diagnosis is confirmed with a Tensilon test, repetitive stimulation in a nerve conduction study, single-fiber EMG, and acetylcholine receptor antibody studies. Treatment includes use of anticholinesterases (e.g., pyridostigmine bromide), steroids, and thymectomy. Sometimes other immunosuppressants, plasmapheresis, or intravenous immunoglobulin are necessary.

9. *Lambert-Eaton syndrome.* This is a rare neuromuscular junction syndrome seen with systemic cancer, especially small-cell cancer of the lung. Proximal weakness and dry mouth are common features. Unlike myasthenia, ocular involvement is rare. Treatment with 4-aminopyridine 3,4-diaminopyridine may be helpful.

Note: The genetics of many hereditary muscle disorders are being established, and previously overlapping syndromes now are recognized to have different genetic sources. The gene for Duchenne muscular dystrophy has been identified, and a protein, dystrophin, appears to play a major role in the disease process. Diagnosis of these conditions in the future may rest on analysis of the genetic makeup of affected patients as much as on the clinical presentation.

Suggested Reading

Amato AA, Barohn RJ. Idiopathic inflammatory myopathies. *Neurol Clin* 1997;15:615–648.

Anagnos A, Ruff RL, Kaminski HJ. Endocrine neuromyopathies. *Neurol Clin* 1997;15:673–696.

Dalakas MC. Polymyositis, dermatomyositis, and inclusion-body myositis. *N Engl J Med* 1991;325:1487–1497.

Drachman DB. Myasthenia gravis. *N Engl J Med* 1994;330:1797–1810.

Gajdos P, Chevret S, Clair B, et al. Clinical trial of plasma exchange and high-dose intravenous immunoglobulin in myasthenia gravis. *Ann Neurol* 1997;41:789–796.

George KK, Pourmand R. Toxic myopathies. *Neurol Clin* 1997;15: 711–730.

Griggs RC, Mendell JR, Miller RG. *Evaluation and treatment of myopathies.* Philadelphia: FA Davis, 1995.

Johnson WG. Friedrich ataxia. *Clin Neurosci* 1995;3:33–38.

Wittbrodt ET. Drugs and myasthenia gravis: an update. *Arch Intern Med* 1997;157:399–408.

Chapter 12

Tremor and Movement Disorders

Case

The wife of a 56-year-old man has noticed that he walks behind her when they go to the park. He seems to have problems getting up from chairs and out of bed. When watching television, his left hand shakes slowly, but this subsides when he uses it. His handwriting has become smaller and difficult to read. His wife constantly has to remind him to "stand up straight." He notices that he has trouble stepping up on a curb, and sometimes he gets stuck in doorways.

Diagnosis

Parkinsonism, probable idiopathic Parkinson's disease.

Tremor involves rhythmic oscillating movement of the extremities or head. Common types of tremor include (a) action tremor of the physiologic, essential, or familial type; (b) intention tremor associated with cerebellar or cerebellar connection disorders; and (c) resting tremor, usually associated with Parkinson's disease. Other movement disorders also are discussed in this chapter.

ACTION TREMOR

Action tremor is a tremor that is most prominent when the limb is held out or being used (action). Patients notice this tremor when holding a coffee cup, writing, or speaking in front of an audience. Such a tremor worsens with anxiety or fatigue. Most people have a mild tremor that may be brought out with caffeine, stimulant medications, or theophylline derivatives. This is known as an exaggerated physiologic tremor. Other medications that may cause such a tremor include valproic acid, lithium, and steroids. Hyperthyroidism, pheochromocytoma, and drug withdrawal also may cause an exaggerated physiologic tremor. Essential tremor is also an action tremor, but it is usually of lower frequency and greater amplitude. Essential tremors may be a genetically determined trait, and some cases run in families (familial action tremor). Essential and familial action tremors tend to gradually worsen over years, particularly when patients reach their 60s. One alcoholic drink will decrease action tremors temporarily. Aside from the tremor, neurologic examination results are normal in such patients. *Note:* Consider Wilson's disease in any young person with an unusual tremor.

Treatment

Physiologic tremor is treated by removing the cause, if possible (stopping drugs or alcohol, treating medical illness, avoiding caffeine). Essential and familial tremors may be suppressed partially by beta blockers, such as propranolol, or by the use of primidone in small doses (25 mg–500 mg/day, titrated slowly). Other medications that may be useful include topiramate and gabapentin. Remember that beta blockers are relatively contraindicated in asthma and congestive heart failure and may cause depression, impotence, and limited exercise tolerance.

INTENTION TREMOR

Intention tremor is not a true tremor but an impairment of the ability to guide limb movements accurately to their destination. An intention tremor is visible when the patient reaches for an object or the examiner's finger. The patient's arm begins to waver from side to side as it nears its goal, as the brain tries to overcorrect for inaccurate movements. Intention tremor is a useful sign of ataxia. Other signs of ataxia include gait incoordination, nystagmus, scanning speech (speech with irregular and choppy phrasing), rebound, and decreased tone. See Chapter 13 for further information on ataxic disorders.

PARKINSONISM

Parkinsonism refers to a complex of alterations of movement that may be caused by Parkinson's disease or other disorders mimicking Parkinson's disease. Features seen in parkinsonism include resting tremor; bradykinesia (decreased movements); rigidity; decreased facial expression; decreased blinking; shuffling gait; and a quiet, hesitant speech pattern (hypophonic). The resting tremor usually consists of a large amplitude, slow (3–7 Hz), "pill-rolling" tremor that is suppressed with movement, as opposed to action tremors that increase with movement. Often there is small handwriting (micrographia) and postural instability.

Parkinson's disease is caused by the degeneration of dopamine-releasing neurons in the substantia nigra of the midbrain. Its three cardinal features are *tremor, bradykinesia, and rigidity*. Decreased dopamine leads to altered activity in the "extrapyramidal" motor system, which leads to the motor abnormalities described. Parkinson's disease is marked pathologically by Lewy bodies and other neuropathologic changes in the remaining neurons of the substantia nigra and other pigmented nuclei of the brainstem.

Differential Diagnosis of Parkinsonism

There are other disorders that may cause parkinsonism besides Parkinson's disease. These may be difficult to separate clinically from Parkinson's disease. Consider the following:

1. *Medications* may cause secondary parkinsonian features, most commonly metoclopramide, major antipsychotic medications, and rarely valproic acid.
2. *Progressive supranuclear palsy* is a degenerative disorder in which patients have a toppling gait, impaired voluntary up-and-down eye movements, and pseudobulbar palsy.
3. *Multiple system atrophy* (MSA) refers to a group of degenerative disorders in which there are signs of other neurologic systems involved, including the corticospinal tract, lower motor neurons, autonomic nervous system, and cerebellum. The Shy-Drager syndrome is a subtype of MSA with impotence, postural hypotension, and parkinsonism. Levodopa is ineffective in this syndrome.

4. *Normal pressure hydrocephalus* involves an early cognitive change and incontinence, particularly following a head injury, subarachnoid hemorrhage, or meningitis. On computed tomography (CT) or magnetic resonance imaging, large ventricles are seen without significant atrophy. Gait is "magnetic," with difficulty picking up the feet despite good strength.

5. A lack of response to adequate antiparkinsonian medication may be a clue to a diagnosis other than Parkinson's disease.

6. Other uncommon neurologic disorders may have symptoms of parkinsonism, including olivopontocerebellar degeneration, striatonigral degeneration (poor response to levodopa), and Wilson's disease (liver dysfunction, Kayser-Fleischer ring).

7. Parkinsonism may be secondary to chronic manganese or carbon monoxide intoxication, MPTP (a "designer" drug), or encephalitis (oculogyric crises).

8. Up to 30% of patients with "typical Parkinson's disease" ultimately are diagnosed at autopsy as having another related disorder.

Treatment of Parkinson's Disease

Treatment of Parkinson's disease has become a specialized endeavor with the continuing development of new medications and treatments. Opinion varies on how to treat early and late disease. The role of surgical intervention is also a continuing issue, and newer surgical approaches may dramatically alter the treatment of this disease in some patients.

Treatment of Early Parkinson's Disease

Patients with early Parkinson's may not require treatment with medication until they experience difficulty functioning. Once difficulty arising from a chair, walking, or using the limbs becomes a problem, medication aimed at improving these functions is indicated.

1. *Amantidine* is an antiviral agent that may improve tremor and bradykinesia early in Parkinson's disease. It blocks reuptake of dopamine into presynaptic neurons and may stimulate postsynaptic receptors. Side effects are mild and include nausea, visual hallucinations, and a mottling of the skin (livido reticularis).

2. *Anticholinergic medications* are helpful for tremor, but their use is limited by side effects. These medications include benztropine mesylate and trihexyphenidyl. Side effects of dry mouth, urinary retention, blurred vision, and confusion are particularly common in elderly patients. Antihistamines are weak antiparkinsonian agents and may be useful.

3. *Levodopa* is the most effective antiparkinsonian medication and is the cornerstone of therapy for most patients. The effect may be dramatic when administered early in disease. Used alone, large doses are needed for effect, and the peripheral effect causes nausea and orthostatic hypotension. When combined with a dopa decarboxylase inhibitor (carbidopa), the peripheral effects are minimized, and the dose may be reduced as more of the dopa reaches the brain to be converted to dopamine. Combination medication is available as short- or long-acting preparation. The short-acting medication is available as 10/100, 25/100, and 25/250, with the first number referring to the milligrams of carbidopa and the second number referring to the milligrams of levodopa. The long-acting (CR) form is available as 25/100 or 50/200 mg. Levodopa/carbidopa 25/100 3 to 4 times a day is the usual starting dose. The most common side effect of levodopa therapy is chorea, with involuntary movements of the face and extremities. Dystonia, agitation, hallucinations, and sleep disorders also may occur, particularly in patients with dementia. Providing levodopa/carbidopa 30 minutes before meals and limiting protein intake during the day may improve absorption and efficacy of levodopa/carbidopa.

4. *Dopamine agonists* are advocated by some authorities as early monotherapy in an attempt to spare the use of levodopa early in the disease, based on the theory that levodopa metabolism byproducts may directly injure the remaining dopaminergic neurons. This theory is controversial. Bromocriptine, pergolide, ropinirole, and pramipexole are the available medications of this type. These medications may help smooth out motor fluctuations with levodopa therapy and have fewer choreiform side effects than levodopa. However, they may cause hypotension, hallucinations, and confusion. Gradual titration to the desired dose is the most effective strategy, and they usually are used in combination with levodopa/carbidopa. A combination of low-dose lev-

odopa/carbidopa and low-dose dopamine agonist commonly is used.

5. *Catecholamine*-O-methyltransferase (COMT) inhibitors extend the pharmacologic half-life of levodopa and may decrease the amount of "off" time.

6. *Selegiline* is a selective monoamine-B oxidase inhibitor that increases the availability of dopamine at the synaptic terminal. A major study (Deprenyl And Tocopherol Antioxidative Therapy Of Parkinsonism, or DATATOP) initially was interpreted as showing a neuroprotective effect of this medication early in Parkinson's disease. Reevaluation of the data showed that the medication has a mild symptomatic effect in early Parkinson's disease. The clinical role of this medication is unclear, and a protective effect has not been proved. Some specialists use selegiline early in Parkinson's disease before instituting other medications.

7. *Domperidone*, where available, is a dopamine receptor antagonist that does not enter the central nervous system and can be used to treat nausea from levodopa and/or dopamine agonists.

Treatment of Late-Stage Parkinson's Disease

After approximately 5 years of treatment with levodopa, probably because of loss of buffering action by remaining dopaminergic neurons, patients develop a variety of difficult-to-treat side effects of levodopa. Such problems include the following:

1. *Wearing-off* of levodopa only a short time after the previous dose. This may be improved by giving the levodopa more frequently, using longer-acting dopa preparations, adding dopamine agonists to levodopa, or adding COMT inhibitors.

2. *Peak-dose dyskinesias* may be helped by using smaller and more frequent levodopa doses or by lowering the levodopa dose and adding dopamine agonists. Long-acting levodopa/carbidopa also may be helpful.

3. "On-off" fluctuations refer to dramatic, unpredictable shifts from undertreated to overtreated states. These are difficult to treat. Liquid levodopa may be helpful, allowing closer dose titration.

4. Confusion, sleep disorder, and psychosis may be helped by decreasing the medication, particularly limiting anticholin-

ergics and amantidine. Adding clozapine or ondansetron may be useful for hallucinations or psychosis.

Note the following when treating patients with Parkinson's disease:

1. It is a progressive disorder, which requires reassessment of mobility issues and caregiver support, and often causes a dependent state.
2. Exercise is useful for patients with Parkinson's disease and should be encouraged.
3. Tricyclic antidepressants can be used for depression in patients receiving levodopa (they may slow absorption via their anticholinergic effects); monoamine oxidase inhibitors are not recommended.
4. Other side effects of levodopa (whether given with or without carbidopa) include postural hypotension (usually asymptomatic) and insomnia.
5. Dementia commonly occurs late in parkinsonism because of concurrent Alzheimer's disease, dementia caused by Parkinson's disease, or diffuse Lewy body disease.
6. Pallidotomy is a new surgical technique in which a lesion is placed in the basal ganglia, which may decrease tremor and levodopa-related dyskinesias. Thalamic and subthalamic nucleus stimulation also may have a beneficial effect on certain aspects of parkinsonism. Patient selection and timing of these procedures are under study.

OTHER MOVEMENT DISORDERS

1. *Tardive dyskinesia* develops in many patients undergoing prolonged treatment with neuroleptic medications, especially the phenothiazines and haloperidol. These movements may persist long after the drug is withdrawn (tardive). Clinically, patients develop an oral–buccal–lingual dyskinesia with involuntary tongue protrusion, lip smacking, and facial grimacing. Occasional involuntary limb and trunk movements occur. Denervation hypersensitivity of brain dopamine receptors may be the cause of tardive dyskinesia. Treatment is difficult and consists primarily of removal of the offending medication, with limited efficacy of medication treatment.

2. *Hemiballismus* is a wild, flinging movement of an entire limb, caused by disease of the subthalamic nucleus and its connections. It is usually a result of infarction in this area of the brain and may be treated with haloperidol or perphenazine. Untreated, it may cause exhaustion and dehydration.

3. *Acute dystonias* include a variety of abnormal postures, usually with turning of the trunk or limbs in uncomfortable, unnatural directions. These may occur as a side effect of neuroleptic drugs, usually in young adults. Treatment with intravenous diphenhydramine (75 mg) or benztropine mesylate (2 mg) usually will reduce these in minutes. In addition to acute dystonia and drug-induced parkinsonism (discussed previously), neuroleptics medications also can cause akathisia (persistent motor restlessness). Chronic dystonia is caused by a variety of inherited disorders and toxins and is outside the scope of this book (see Suggested Reading).

4. *Myoclonus*, or shocklike, nonpatterned contractions of a muscle or group of muscles, often occurs in a variety of muscle groups (multifocal myoclonus). They occur in a variety of disorders, including anoxia, myoclonic epilepsies, and some degenerative disorders such as Creutzfeldt-Jakob disease. They also can be seen in metabolic encephalopathies (particularly with uremia) and certain drug intoxications (e.g., imipramine toxicity). Drugs useful in treatment include clonazepam, valproic acid, and 5-hydroxytryptophan.

5. *Chorea* refers to involuntary, irregular, jerky movements of various body parts, resembling restlessness. Choreic movements are seen in Parkinson's disease with dopa therapy, Huntington's disease, Sydenham's chorea, and lupus erythematosus, in association with pregnancy (chorea gravidarum), and in some children with cerebral palsy. Patients with *athetosis* have slow writhing movement of the fingers and hands.

6. *Tics* are erratic, coordinated, stereotyped, irresistible behaviors. Some are motor (sudden jerk of the head, shoulder movement, clapping, obscene gestures), whereas others are vocal (snorts, sniffing, occasionally involuntary obscene speech). An obsessive-compulsive disorder often coexists with the tics. Tics may be inherited as part of a symptom complex in the *Gilles de la Tourette's* syndrome.

Suggested Reading

Albanese A, Colosimo C, Bentivoglio AR, et al. Multiple system atrophy presenting as parkinsonism. *J Neurol Neurosurg Psychiatr* 1995;59: 144–151.

Anouti A, Koller WC. Tremor disorders. *West J Med* 1995;162:510–513.

Caparros-Lefebvre D, Blond S, Vermersch P, et al. Chronic thalamic stimulation improves tremor and levodopa-induced dyskinesias in Parkinson's disease. *J Neurol Neurosurg Psychiatr* 1993;56:268–273.

Caviness JN. Myoclonus. *Mayo Clin Proc* 1996;71:679–688.

Daniel SE, de Bruin VM, Lees AJ. The clinical and pathological spectrum of Steele-Richardson-Olszewski syndrome (progressive supranuclear palsy): a reappraisal. *Brain* 1995;118:759–770.

Dystonia. In: Fahn S, Marsden CD, Calne DB, eds. *Advances in neurology,* Vol 50. New York: Raven Press, 1988.

Guttman M, Kish SJ, Furukawa Y. Current concepts in the diagnosis and management of Parkinson's disease. *CMAJ* 2003;168:293–301.

Lozano AM, Lang AE, Galvez-Jimenez N, et al. Effect of GPi pallidotomy on motor function in Parkinson's disease. *Lancet* 1995;346: 1383–1387.

Nutt JG, Marsden CD, Thompson PD. Human walking and higher-level gait disorders, particularly in the elderly. *Neurology* 1993;43:268–279.

Stern M. Contemporary approaches to the pharmacotherapeutic management of Parkinson's disease: an overview. *Neurology* 1997;49 (suppl 1):S2–S9.

Waters CH. Managing the late complications of Parkinson's disease. *Neurology* 1997;49(suppl 1):S57.

Chapter 13

Ataxia

Ataxia is a disorder of coordination and rhythm. Because many parts of the nervous system participate in carrying out coordinated movements, ataxia may result from anatomic dysfunction at different levels of the neuraxis. Localizing ataxia is key in establishing the cause. In this chapter, ataxia is classified anatomically and some of the common causes are discussed.

Signs of ataxia include the following:

1. Intention tremor
2. Unsteady gait, often with a wide base
3. Dysdiadochokinesia: when alternately supinating and pronating the hand, there are slow, irregular, and arrhythmic movements
4. Overshoot dysmetria: the patient often launches a limb to the target, overshoots, and then recorrects. This is the basis of intention tremor.
5. Nystagmus

IS THE LESION IN THE FRONTAL LOBE?

[Mechanism: involvement of corticocerebellar connections (i.e., frontopontocerebellar pathway)].

1. *Tumor.* Meningioma, glioma, or metastatic tumor may involve the frontal lobes. Patients may have signs suggesting cerebellar disease (i.e., staggering gait, difficulty performing rapid alternating movements, and even nystagmus). Patients with "frontal ataxia" tend to fall backward. Other features of

frontal lobe dysfunction include perseveration, grasp and primitive suck reflexes, incontinence, slowness in thinking and initiating conversation, and headache.

2. *Anterior cerebral artery syndrome.* A thrombotic occlusion of this artery affects the frontal lobes (see Chapter 16). A large aneurysm of the anterior communicating artery also may affect the frontal lobes.

3. *Hydrocephalus.* Enlargement of the frontal horns of the lateral ventricles affects leg fibers and may produce ataxia. In addition, there is memory loss and incontinence. Hydrocephalus may occur with tumors that obstruct the ventricular system or with disorders of cerebrospinal fluid (CSF) absorption (see Chapter 31).

IS THE LESION SUBCORTICAL?

(Mechanism: involvement of corticocerebellar connections, plus pyramidal tract dysfunction.)

1. *Multiple strokes* (état lacunaire). In addition to ataxia, there is emotional lability, brisk reflexes including increased jaw jerk, dysarthria, and dementia (see Chapter 19).

2. *Ataxic hemiparesis.* This is a lacunar syndrome with the lesion in the internal capsule or contralateral basis pontis. There is ataxia on the same side as the hemiparesis, with weakness primarily in the leg.

IS THE LESION IN THE THALAMUS?

[Mechanism: involvement of ventral lateral (VL) nucleus and adjacent subthalamic region.] Occasionally, patients with thalamic infarction may develop a sensory ataxia, with incoordination based on a profound loss of position sense. This will be unilateral, affecting arm and leg. Check for sensory loss in any patient with ataxia. Lesions in the dentatorubrothalamic projection to the VL nucleus of the thalamus result in hemiataxia of the contralateral limbs.

IS THE LESION IN THE BRAINSTEM?

(Mechanism: involvement of cerebellar connections.) The two most common causes of ataxia secondary to brainstem lesions are stroke and multiple sclerosis. Diagnosis is based on history and findings of other brainstem signs (e.g., crossed motor or sensory findings, internuclear ophthalmoplegia, nystagmus, dysarthria).

IS THE LESION IN THE CEREBELLUM?

(Mechanism: direct involvement of coordination pathways.)

1. *Signs.* Signs of cerebellar dysfunction include limb, trunk, gait, and speech ataxia; nystagmus; and hypotonia. Depending on whether midline or lateral cerebellar structures are involved, there may or may not be limb ataxia or prominent gaze-evoked nystagmus. Midline cerebellar lesions produce truncal and gait ataxia. Cerebellar hemisphere lesions characteristically cause limb ataxia and nystagmus. An impaired checking response (unable to halt sudden movements) may be present. A subtle cerebellar disorder may be detected by problems with tandem gait (walking with one foot in front of the other). *Note: Cerebellar hemispheric lesions cause ipsilateral ataxia.*

2. *Cerebellar hemorrhage, infarct, tumor.* These usually are associated occipital headache and ocular gaze palsies. Limb strength and sensation are preserved. *Remember the need for emergency computed tomography scan for diagnosis and often the need for surgical intervention* (see Chapter 16). Primary cerebellar tumors are seen in childhood; they are rare in adults. Metastatic tumors often involve the cerebellum in adults.

3. *Spinocerebellar degeneration.* These syndromes include olivopontocerebellar degeneration and Friedreich's ataxia. In Friedreich's ataxia, there is usually a positive family history, a chronic course, and evidence of more widespread nervous system involvement, such as peripheral neuropathy (loss of reflexes) and pyramidal tract dysfunction (up-going toes). Pes cavus (high arched feet) or scoliosis sometimes is associated with these degenerations.

4. *Alcoholism* or occult malignancy. These may be associated with cerebellar degeneration. Alcoholic cerebellar degeneration is characterized by ataxia of gait and of the legs, with less prominent involvement of arms, speech, or ocular motility. There is usually an associated memory loss and polyneuropathy. Acute ataxia and oculomotor paralysis associated with alcoholism (Wernicke's encephalopathy) respond to thiamine administration (see Chapter 27).

5. *Occult malignancy.* This may have cerebellar ataxia as a presenting symptom, especially carcinoma of the breast or ovary. Check for anti Yo antibodies in serum or CSF.
6. *Acute cerebellitis.* This is a viral or postviral cause of ataxia seen in children and rarely in adults.

IS THE LESION IN THE SPINAL CORD?

(Mechanism: ataxia through posterior column dysfunction, involvement of pyramidal tracts.) Remember, a positive Romberg sign (unsteady with eyes closed, steady with eyes open) usually indicates posterior column disease. Magnetic resonance imaging (MRI) is usually diagnostic.

1. Patients with *cervical spondylosis* with associated cervical myelopathy usually have neck and arm pain and abnormal cervical spine films. Depending on the extent of spinal cord involvement, there may be posterior column dysfunction and up-going toes (pyramidal tract involvement).
2. *Multiple sclerosis* often involves the spinal cord. Diagnosis is made on the basis of finding multiple lesions of the nervous system (e.g., optic neuritis, brainstem signs), a history of attacks, elevation of CSF gamma globulin, and an abnormal brain MRI.
3. *Vitamin B$_{12}$ deficiency* may produce subacute combined degeneration, with involvement of the lateral and posterior columns of the spinal cord. Ataxia is based on a combination of weakness and position sense loss. Often there is also a peripheral neuropathy making the interpretation of physical signs more difficult.
4. Other causes of ataxia secondary to spinal cord dysfunction include spinal cord tumor and tabes dorsalis

IS THE LESION IN PERIPHERAL NERVE?

(Mechanism: ataxia secondary to weakness or loss of position sense.)

1. *Miller-Fisher syndrome* is an acute syndrome characterized by gait ataxia, loss of deep tendon reflexes, and ophthalmoparesis. It is a variant of Guillain-Barré syndrome.
2. Ataxia also may be a feature of severe *peripheral neuropathies* from other causes (sensory ataxia). Some patients develop a

sensory ataxia from degeneration of the dorsal root ganglia, a ganglioneuritis. This can be seen with remote neoplasms (paraneoplastic neuropathy), Sjögren's syndrome, or chemotherapy or as an idiopathic disorder.
3. Occasionally, early in Guillain-Barré syndrome, gait ataxia may precede frank muscle weakness and reflex loss.

IS THE LESION IN MUSCLE?

Muscle disorders usually present with weakness rather than ataxia.

CHRONIC CAUSES OF ATAXIA

Rarer causes of chronic progressive ataxia include Friedreich's ataxia, Charcot-Marie-Tooth disease, Ramsey Hunt syndrome, familial spastic ataxia, and Huntington's disease.

ACUTE CAUSES OF ATAXIA

Acute ataxia occurs in acute cerebellitis, drug and chemical ingestion, acute labyrinthitis, lupus erythematosus, and stroke syndrome. The time course differentiates acute from chronic ataxia.

Suggested Reading

Bolla L, Palmer RM. Paraneoplastic cerebellar degeneration. Case report and literature review. *Arch Intern Med* 1997;157:1258–1262.

Gilman S, Newman S. *Manter and Gatz's essentials of clinical neuroanatomy and neurophysiology,* 7th ed. Philadelphia: FA Davis, 1987.

Koeppen AH. The hereditary ataxias. *J Neuropathol Exp Neurol* 1998:57: 531–543.

Chapter 14

Sleep Disorders

Case

A 56-year-old man who weighs 343 pounds complains that he often awakens fatigued and with a headache and must nap throughout the day to continue working. His wife has no idea whether he sleeps because she moved to another room years ago to avoid his heavy snoring. He sometimes would stop breathing for a few seconds and then begin again with a snort. He has been visiting a cardiologist for an unexplained arrhythmia.

Diagnosis

Obstructive Sleep Apnea

Sleep disorders are more common than generally realized. Approximately 10% to 15% of the population has sleep-related problems. Early diagnosis and proper treatment depend on an awareness of characteristic symptoms. Sleep disorders are separated into three groups:

- Disorders of excessive somnolence (DOES), such as narcolepsy and sleep apnea
- Disorders of initiation and maintenance of sleep (DIMS), such as insomnia
- Abnormal behaviors caused by sleep disorders (parasomnias), such as sleepwalking and night terrors

Take a sleep history from the patient *and* the bed partner:

1. When does the patient go to bed? How long until the patient falls asleep? Does the patient wake up at night? When does the patient awaken in the morning?
2. What medications or stimulants do the patient take? What beverages do the patient drink? What activities are done before going to bed?
3. Does the patient toss and turn (unrestorative sleep)? Are there sudden jerking leg movements ("periodic leg movements")?
4. Does the patient feel the urge to move the legs from time to time (restless leg syndrome)? Is there loud snoring, or are there long pauses between breaths (sleep apnea)?
5. Does the patient have unusual activities at night, such as sleep-walking or violent dreams (parasomnias)?
6. Does the patient wake up feeling refreshed, even after a short nap (narcolepsy)?

Examination results of patients with sleep disorders are usually normal except for body habitus. Middle-aged patients with sleep apnea frequently are obese men with thick necks. Sometimes enlarged tonsils, adenoids, or other pharyngeal abnormalities can contribute to obstructive sleep apnea, as can micrognathia (jaw abnormalities). Altered or narrowed nasal passages also may cause obstructive sleep apnea. Search for signs of hypothyroidism or acromegaly, which may be associated with sleep disorders. Note the presence of hypertension or cardiomegaly.

DISORDERS OF EXCESSIVE SOMNOLENCE (DOES)

Manifestations of excessive sleepiness or drowsiness during the day include falling asleep during activities such as eating, driving, or sitting in a class. Causes include situational sleep deprivation (e.g., students who stay awake too late, parents with small children), use of certain medications or intoxicants (e.g., sedatives, antidepressants, muscle relaxants, ethanol), depression (may decrease or increase sleep time), or disorders of sleep such as narcolepsy or sleep apnea.

Narcolepsy

In narcolepsy, a genetically determined disorder, patients have one or more of the following:

1. *Sleep attacks*: uncontrollable attacks of sleep for short periods
2. *Cataplexy*: sudden loss of muscle tone, induced by emotion or sudden stimuli
3. *Sleep paralysis*: at waking or in transition to sleep, the patient is unable to move
4. *Hypnagogic hallucinations*: vivid dreamlike hallucinations just before falling asleep or when just awakening
5. *Automatic behavior*: attention lapses in which routine activities are continued and the patient is amnesic for the behavior

Sleep Apnea

In sleep apnea, the patient may have one or more of the following: restless sleep, enuresis, impotence, morning headaches, memory disturbances, learning problems, heavy snoring, or hypertension. Seizure disorders and headache disorders may be worsened by sleep apnea.

1. *Obstructive sleep apnea* is a condition in which patients have respiratory movements in sleep, but excessive weight or an abnormal oropharynx make these ineffective. The consequence is snoring and episodes of breathing cessation. Oxygenation decreases during the episodes, and sleep often is disrupted. Hypertension, polycythemia, arrhythmias, and cor pulmonale may occur if sleep apnea is untreated.
2. *Central sleep apnea* has been observed with a variety of neurologic disorders that disrupt the lower brainstem. Here, episodes of apnea are unaccompanied by respiratory movements. Central sleep apnea is much less common than obstructive sleep apnea. Patients may have a combination of obstructive and central sleep apnea.

DISORDERS OF INITIATION AND MAINTENANCE OF SLEEP (DIMS)

The patient with insomnia cannot fall asleep at night, has difficulty staying asleep, and/or wakes up early. Disturbed nocturnal sleep leads to daytime drowsiness. Consider the following:

1. Does the patient participate in stimulating activities before sleep, such as exercise, paying the bills, or in some instances, watching television?

2. Are there symptoms of depression, including poor appetite, early awakening, weight loss, or sadness, suggesting a secondary sleep disorder?

3. Does the patient have chronic renal failure or alcoholism, each of which has been associated with secondary sleep disorders?

4. Are there symptoms of anxiety that are disturbing sleep, or are there other psychiatric abnormalities ?

5. Does the patient take certain medications, such as caffeine, stimulants, and certain antidepressants, which may cause secondary insomnia?

PARASOMNIAS

In parasomnias, abnormal behaviors occur in association with sleep disorders.

1. *Sleepwalking* is common, usually is seen in childhood, and may suggest a psychiatric disorder or medication intoxication if it begins in adulthood.

2. *Body jerks and sensory symptoms* while falling asleep are common and usually benign.

3. *Paroxysmal bursts* of choreoathetoid movements in sleep (*nocturnal paroxysmal dystonia*) may respond to antiepileptic drugs.

4. *Night terrors* are common in childhood. Children awaken with fright, tachycardia, and inconsolable distress for a few minutes. Children tend to outgrow this condition.

5. *Violent behavior* in rapid eye movement (REM) sleep may occur in older males and may be dangerous to the patient and bed partner if left untreated. Some of these patients develop parkinsonism.

6. Seizures may occur in sleep and may be difficult to separate from nonepileptic parasomnias.

LABORATORY EVALUATION

In narcolepsy, the results of a sleep electroencephalogram (EEG) combined with electromyographic (EMG) and electrooculographic monitoring (a polysomnogram) are frequently abnormal, showing REM sleep at sleep outset rather than later in the sleep cycle. Results of a multiple sleep latency test, which measures the time to fall asleep (latency), are usually abnormal. In sleep apnea, a record of the patient's breathing pattern during sleep is necessary. Monitoring O_2, respiratory efforts, and electrocardiogram can help distinguish between obstructive, central, or mixed types of sleep apnea. Periodic leg movements can be recorded by monitoring EMG activity of the legs during sleep. Parasomnias are recorded by a combination of EEG and video monitoring in the setting of a sleep study. These studies are best performed in laboratories with particular interest and expertise in sleep disorders.

TREATMENT

1. *Sleep apnea*: Weight loss; treatment with respiratory stimulants; tonsillectomy; palatopharyngoplasty; and, if necessary, tracheostomy may be indicated in the treatment of obstructive sleep apnea. Continuous positive airway pressure at night may prove helpful in treatment and reduces awakenings and daytime sleepiness. Stimulants and rarely diaphragmatic pacing are used in the central type.
2. *Narcolepsy*: Frequent naps and judicious use of stimulant drugs, such as pemoline and methylphenidate, are helpful in narcolepsy. Modafinil is chemically distinct from the stimulant drugs and is useful in narcolepsy. Tricyclic antidepressants, such as protriptyline and clomipramine, are useful in cataplexy. Selective serotonin reuptake inhibitors also may be used for cataplexy.
3. *Insomnia*: The treatment of insomnia is difficult and must be tailored to the individual patient. Modalities include environmental manipulation (e.g., altering bedtime routine, doing a relaxing evening exercise, taking a hot bath before sleep), relaxation techniques, psychotherapy, and short-term hypnotic drug use. Remember, elderly patients normally require less sleep than when they were younger.
4. Useful tips for patients with insomnia:
   - Reserve bed for sleeping and sex (i.e., no eating, reading, watching television, or tossing and turning).
   - Go to sleep at the same time every night, and get up at the same time every morning.

- Do not eat large meals before bed.
- Do not consume alcohol as a hypnotic.
- If unable to sleep after a fixed amount of time (e.g., 40 minutes), get up and do something else.
- Turn the clock around so you cannot see it; there is no value in being aware of how late it is when you cannot sleep.

Suggested Reading

Aldrich MS. Narcolepsy. *N Engl J Med* 1990;323:389–395.

Barthlen GM. Sleep disorders. Obstructive sleep apnea, restless legs syndrome, and insomnia in geriatric patients. *Geriatrics* 2002;57:34–39.

Chesson AL, Ferber RA, Fry JM, et al. The indications for polysomnography and related procedures. *Sleep* 1997;20:423–487.

Mahowald MW, Schenck CH. NREM sleep parasomnias. *Neurol Clin* 1996;14:675–696.

Printz PN, Vitiello MV, Raskind MA, et al. Geriatrics: sleep disorders and aging. *N Engl J Med* 1990;323:520–526.

Schenck CH, Bundlie SR, Mahowald MW. Delayed emergence of parkinsonian disorder in 38% of 29 older men initially diagnosed with idiopathic rapid eye movement sleep behavior disorder. *Neurology* 1996;46:388–393.

Schenck CH, Mahowald MW. REM sleep parasomnias. *Neurol Clin* 1996;14:697–720.

Silber MH. Sleep disorders. *Neurol Clin* 2001;19:173–186.

Spielman AJ, Nunes J, Glovinsky PB. Insomnia. *Neurol Clin* 1996;14: 513–543.

Stollo PJ, Rogers RM. Obstructive sleep apnea. *N Engl J Med* 1996;334: 99–104.

Trenkwalder C, Walters AS, Hening W. Periodic limb movements and restless leg syndrome. *Neurol Clin* 1996;14:629–650.

U.S. Modafinil in Narcolepsy Multicenter Study Group. Randomized trial of modafinil for the treatment of pathological somnolence in narcolepsy. *Ann Neurol* 1998;43:88–97.

Chapter 15

Stroke

Case

A 67-year-old man with diabetes, longstanding hypertension, and a pack-a-day smoking habit presents to the emergency room 45 minutes after suddenly dropping his fork from his right hand at lunch. His wife noticed he was using the wrong words and had trouble understanding her, and he had to be assisted to the ambulance because of right leg weakness. In the emergency room, he shows signs of a global aphasia, right hemiparesis affecting the arm and face more than the leg, and moderate hypertension. A computed tomography (CT) scan shows no evidence of hemorrhage or cerebral edema. He is considered for thrombolytic therapy.

Diagnosis

Cerebral infarction in left hemisphere caused by embolus or thrombosis in the middle cerebral artery territory.

Stroke is one of the most common neurologic problems and the third leading cause of death in the United States. Despite considerable advances, some aspects of the treatment of stroke remain controversial. This chapter presents a basic approach to the patient with stroke and outlines generally accepted therapy. Therapy of stroke is evolving with the introduction of newer medications and interventions.

TABLE 15.1.   Stroke Types

Infarction
  Thrombotic
    Large vessel
    Small vessel (lacunar stroke)
  Embolic
Hemorrhage
  Intracerebral
    Deep
    Lobar
  Subarachnoid
  Subdural
  Epidural

STROKE TYPES

Stroke is a general term for the sudden onset of a focal neurologic deficit caused by vascular disease. There are subcategories
of stroke, each with a specific cause, course, and treatment
(Table 15.1). Infarction refers to stroke in which there is a loss of
blood supply to part of the brain, so that ischemic injury occurs.
Infarction may be thrombotic (i.e., caused by blood clot formation within a vessel) or embolic (caused by material formed proximally, such as at a heart valve or carotid plaque, and then dis-
lodged to occlude a distal vessel). Thrombotic stroke often is
characterized as large vessel (e.g., carotid, vertebral, or basilar
arteries) or small vessel (e.g., the lenticulostriate branches of the
middle cerebral artery). Hemorrhage may be intracerebral (in
the brain parenchyma) or surrounding the brain (subarachnoid,
subdural, or epidural).

WHERE IS THE STROKE? WHAT IS THE ANATOMY?

1. Intracerebral hemorrhage is usually deep in the brain and
   may affect the putamen, thalamus, cerebellum, or pons.
   Lobar hemorrhages also occur.
2. Emboli tend to produce superficial wedge-shaped infarcts as
   a result of the distal migration of emboli, giving cortical
   deficits or deficits at the top of the basilar artery territory.
3. Thrombosis produces a variety of syndromes with the diagnosis based on history, anatomy of the lesion, mechanism of
   the thrombosis, and exclusion of embolic or hemorrhagic

strokes. Any part of the brain or brainstem may be involved in thrombotic stroke.

4. Lacunar strokes usually involve the deep white matter, basal ganglia, or brainstem. The small, well-circumscribed lesions may give characteristic clinical symptoms and signs that strongly suggest the diagnosis of lacunar disease (see Chapter 16).

5. Subarachnoid hemorrhage causes sudden and severe headache and stiff neck, and may also cause symptoms at the hemorrhage site (e.g., anterior communicating artery: mutism and paraparesis). Often there is no focal neurologic deficit.

HOW DID THE STROKE DEVELOP?

1. Intracranial hemorrhage occurs during waking hours, usually in a known hypertensive patient or in a patient with a bleeding tendency (e.g., a patient receiving anticoagulant medication). The full deficit seldom is present at onset but develops gradually over minutes to hours. There rarely is a warning; headache, nausea, and vomiting are usually, but not invariably, present.

2. Emboli usually give a maximal deficit at onset and often occur during waking hours. The deficit may improve in hours. There may be headache or focal seizures.

3. Thrombosis often occurs during sleep or is present on awakening. Symptoms and signs usually progress in a stepwise fashion; it may take hours or days for the full deficit to develop. A warning is common in thrombotic strokes. The patient may have a headache and frequently has a history of prior transient ischemic attacks (TIAs), which are brief episodes of neurologic symptoms resulting from vascular disease (see Chapter 17).

4. Lacunar or small-vessel thrombotic strokes occur either abruptly or in a stuttering course over hours or days. There may be warning TIAs, but headache is uncommon. There are usually risk factors such as hypertension or diabetes.

5. Subarachnoid hemorrhage occurs abruptly with a severe "worst headache of my life" as the cardinal feature. Onset is often during exertion, with an associated stiff neck and photophobia. A "sentinal" headache may occur days or weeks prior to a major subarachnoid hemorrhage.

WHAT ARE HISTORICAL CLUES AND PHYSICAL FINDINGS?

Is There Evidence for Occlusion or Stenosis of Internal or Common Carotid Artery?

1. One of the most common causes of TIA or stroke is athero-sclerotic disease affecting the internal carotid artery at its origin, with stroke occurring as a result of thrombosis of the vessel or embolism to distal branches of the internal carotid.

2. Clinical signs may include a carotid bruit (most significant if high pitched and at the angle of the jaw), contralateral ocular bruit, or a decreased pulsation of the carotid in the neck. Horner's syndrome may be seen ipsilateral to a carotid occlusion or dissection.

3. Occasionally, atheromatous emboli (Hollenhorst plaques) to the retinal arteries may be seen on funduscopic examination on the same side as a carotid stenosis.

    Note: A carotid bruit does not prove carotid stenosis; absence of a bruit does not rule out stenosis. Studies to determine the degree of carotid stenosis are necessary.

4. In addition to the physical examination of the carotids, there are noninvasive tests. Such tests, including duplex carotid ultrasound and transcranial Doppler (TCD), may be helpful to identify and characterize carotid lesions. Each of these tests assesses different aspects of cerebrovascular flow and anatomy and may be used to determine the degree of stenosis and abnormalities of carotid flow (Table 15.2).

TABLE 15.2. Cerebrovascular Disorders that Cause Stroke

Atherosclerosis
Embolism
Aneurysm
Fibromuscular dysplasia
Arteriovenous malformation
Hypercoagulable states
    Fever/infection
    Postoperative state
    Antiphospholipid antibodies, rarer hypercoagulable states
    Estrogen use
Trauma, vascular dissection
Vasculitis, central nervous system infection
Sickle cell anemia
Drug use
Bleeding diatheses (anticoagulant use, hemophilia, etc.)

Magnetic resonance angiography (MRA) may also be useful in assessing carotid stenosis. A combination of noninvasive vascular testing and imaging are supplanting conventional angiography in preoperative assessment for carotid endarterectomy. CT angiography (CTa) is another technique that is useful in showing stenosis in extracranial and intracranial vessels.

Large- or Small-Vessel Disease?

Warning symptoms tend to be stereotyped in small-vessel disease and occur over hours to days. In large-vessel disease, the symptoms frequently vary depending on which territory of the vessel is involved during the warning; symptoms usually precede the stroke by days or weeks but may occur over a period of months. See Table 15.2 for cerebrovascular diseases that cause stroke.

Headache is common with large-vessel occlusion. Posterior circulation stroke often produces headache over the occiput, and anterior circulation stroke usually produces headache behind the eyes or over the forehead or temples. Headache rarely accompanies small-vessel occlusion.

Is There an Embolic Focus?

The heart is the most common source of emboli, although emboli may arise from a plaque in a diseased carotid artery or aorta. Cardiogenic emboli account for 15% to 20% of all ischemic strokes. Cardiac factors predisposing to emboli include mural thrombi, especially with anterior wall myocardial infarction (MI) and left-ventricular wall abnormality (emboli usually occur within 10 days but sometimes months after the MI and may be the presenting feature of an MI), mitral valve disease, or atrial fibrillation. Transesophageal echocardiography is proving to be valuable in more clearly imaging cardiac abnormalities that serve as potential sources of stroke. These include mural thrombus, atrial septal defects, atrial septal aneurysms, patent foramen ovale, and atherosclerotic plaques in the ascending aorta. Paroxysmal cardiac arrhythmias are an important cause of embolic stroke and may require a Holter monitor for detection. Atrial fibrillation is a major independent risk factor for stroke, whether persistent or paroxysmal. Other cardiac embolic risk factors include prosthetic or calcified valves, bacterial endocarditis, marantic endocarditis, atrial myxoma, and nonischemic cardiomyopathies.

Is There a Coagulation Deficit or Systemic Cause of Stroke?

Stroke may occur in the absence of vascular disease, cardiac source, or trauma. In such cases, a coagulation deficit may be the underlying mechanism. Hypercoagulable states may occur during surgery, infection, or pregnancy. A variety of familial coagulation deficits that predispose to thrombosis are known, such as protein C and S deficiencies, antithrombin III deficiency, sickle cell anemia, and factor V Leiden. Homocystinuria and hyperhomocystinemia cause accelerated atherosclerosis. The lupus anticoagulant and antiphospholipid antibodies may be important risk factors in strokes in the young and in patients without lupus erythematosus or other collagen vascular disorders. Drug and alcohol abuse is associated with a variety of strokes, both thrombotic and hemorrhagic.

Is There an Intracranial Hemorrhage?

1. The diagnosis of subarachnoid hemorrhage is usually apparent from the history and physical examination. A noncontrast CT scan is often diagnostic, but in approximately 5% of cases, the CT is negative. In such cases, a lumbar puncture is important because it may show bloody cerebrospinal fluid (CSF), elevated pressure, increased protein, or xanthochromia (a yellowish tinge of the CSF caused by red blood cell breakdown). If subarachnoid hemorrhage has occurred, four-vessel angiography will help in locating the source of bleeding, most typically from an intracranial berry aneurysm (approximately 20% of such aneurysms are multiple). CTa or MRA can identify larger aneurysms, but neither is the "gold-standard" for diagnosis. In patients with a subarachnoid bleed and a negative angiogram, magnetic resonance imaging (MRI) may show thrombus inside an aneurysm, avoiding misdiagnosis.

2. Intracerebral hemorrhage is usually evident on the CT or MRI scan and is suspected clinically by progressive deficit over hours or minutes and the presence of decreased consciousness, both of which are common in this disorder. The most common causes of nontraumatic intracerebral hemorrhage are hypertension and trauma. Other causes include blood dyscrasias, anticoagulants, drug abuse (cocaine or

amphetamines), amyloid angiopathy, brain tumors, and arteriovenous malformations (AVMs).

3. The diagnosis of subdural or epidural hemorrhage usually is based on the history of recent trauma to the head, with CT scan or MRI confirming the diagnosis. Noncontrast CT may miss small subdural hematomas.

Note: It is important to realize that there are exceptions to these rules. Embolic stroke can progress in a stepwise fashion, thrombosis can occur during the day, and hemorrhage may masquerade as thrombosis. Nevertheless, these rules are useful; when combined with other information about the patient, they help lead to the diagnosis. See Table 15.3 for characteristic features of stroke.

Stroke in Young Adults

When evaluating stroke in young adults, pursue risk factors such as use of oral contraceptives, previously undetected hypertension, mitral valve prolapse, patent foramen ovale with paradoxic embolism, hypercoagulable states, and metabolic disorders (e.g., homocystinuria).

Cocaine abuse, binge or high alcohol consumption, and smoking are important causes of stroke in the young adult. Stroke syndromes associated with cocaine include subarachnoid hemorrhage caused by rupture of aneurysms and AVMs, intracerebral hemorrhage, and cerebral infarction. Excessive alcohol consumption is associated with hypertension, intracranial hemorrhage, cerebral infarction, and increased risk of death from stroke. Abuse of amphetamine has been associated with intracranial hemorrhage ("speed" hemorrhage). Therefore, ask about drug and alcohol use in these patients and obtain a drug screen.

Arterial dissection is an important cause of stroke in young adults and often is heralded by sharp pain in the neck. It may result from trauma, neck exercise, or cervical manipulation, although often it is spontaneous. Imaging with MRA or CTa is usually diagnostic.

Laboratory Investigation

Laboratory investigation of the stroke patient should include the following:

TABLE 15.3. Characteristic Features of Stroke[a]

	Embolus	Large Vessel Thrombosis	Lacune	Intracerebral Hemorrhage	Subarachnoid Hemorrhage
Location	Peripheral (cortical)	Variable (depends on vessel)	Pons, internal capsule	Deep (basal ganglia, thalamus, cerebellum)	Vessels at junction of the circle of Willis
Onset	Sudden (maximum deficit at onset)	Sudden, gradual, stepwise, or stuttering	Sudden, gradual, stepwise, or stuttering	Sudden (deficit develops over minutes to hours)	Sudden, usually few or no focal signs
When	Awake	Asleep or inactive	Asleep or inactive	Awake and active	Awake and active
Warning (TIA)	None	Usually	Variable, TIAs may occur	None	Variable, occasionally sentinel headache
Headache	Sometimes	Sometimes	No	Usually	Always (stiff neck)
CT scan	Decreased density	Decreased density	Decreased density	Increased density	Usually normal
MRI T_1	Hypointense	Hypointense	Usually normal	b	Usually normal[a]
MRI T_2	Hyperintense	Hyperintense	Hyperintense	b	Usually normal[a]
LP	Usually clear	Clear	Clear	Usually bloody[c]	Invariably bloody

CT, computed tomography; LP, lumbar puncture; MRI, magnetic resonance imaging; TIA, transient ischemic attack.

[a]These characteristics are generally accepted principles regarding stroke; however, remember they are not hard rules and stroke can present atypically.

[b]The appearance of hemorrhage on MRI scan is variable and depends on multiple factors, such as type of scan (T_1 versus T_2 weighted), location (intraparenchymal versus extradural versus subarachnoid), and time (acute, subacute, chronic).

[c]Note: LP not recommended in intracerebral hemorrhage.

- *Complete blood count*: blood dyscrasia, polycythemia, thrombocytopenia, thrombocytosis, or infection (neutrophilia) as risk factors for stroke
- *Prothrombin time, partial thromboplastin time*: clue to the patient with antiphospholipid antibody (prolonged partial thromboplastin time) or other coagulopathy
- *Urinalysis*: hematuria in subacute bacterial endocarditis (SBE) with embolic stroke
- *Sedimentation rate*: elevation a clue to vasculitis, hyperviscosity, or SBE as cause of stroke
- *Chemistry screen*: elevation a clue to vasculitis, hyperviscosity, or SBE as cause of stroke
- *Chest radiograph*: enlarged heart as embolic source of stroke or evidence of prolonged hypertension; may detect an unsuspected malignancy
- *Electrocardiogram*: may reveal arrhythmia, recent myocardial infarct, or enlarged left atrium as a source of embolism
- *Risk factor screen*: lipid profile, hemoglobin A1c, homocysteine

Cranial Computerized Tomography

The CT scan is useful in separating hemorrhagic (intracerebral or subarachnoid hemorrhage) from nonhemorrhagic (thrombotic or embolic) stroke. Blood present in a fresh hemorrhage produces an area of increased density; infarction produces an area of decreased density. In addition, the CT scan may help to define the location and size of the lesion (e.g., cortical versus subcortical infarctions), as well as small-vessel versus large-vessel disease.

1. The CT scan is positive in virtually all cases of intracerebral hemorrhage (increased density) and often shows interhemispheric blood or bleeding into brain parenchyma in subarachnoid hemorrhage. These changes are evident within the first hour after onset of symptoms. With CT scanning, patients with the clinical diagnosis of thrombosis often have intracerebral hemorrhage.
2. The CT scan is positive in most cases of cerebral infarction (decreased density), but these changes may only be evident 24 to 48 hours after the onset of symptoms. With contrast enhancement, infarcts may mimic tumors on CT scan, but the enhancement is generally not associated with the signifi-

cant mass effect that occurs with enhancement of brain tumors. In some instances, a mass effect may be present with infarction, raising the question of a brain tumor; MRI, serial CT scans, and clinical observation will clarify the diagnosis.

3. A hemorrhagic infarct is often secondary to a large embolus. This produces increased density in CT scan. Anticoagulation should be delayed initially when hemorrhage is associated with embolic infarction.

4. Brainstem hemorrhage is usually visible on CT scan, but brainstem infarction may not be visible because of bony artifact at the base of the skull.

5. The CT scan identifies major shifts of intracranial contents that may require aggressive medical and surgical measures to control edema (see Chapter 31).

6. Subdural hematomas may be recognized on CT scan by shifts of intracranial contents, partial obliteration of a lateral ventricle or of sulci, and changes in density (depending on the age of the lesion) on the surface of the brain.

7. Brain tumors are identified on CT scan by characteristic density patterns, contrast enhancement, and mass effects. A small percentage of brain tumors present clinically as strokes.

Magnetic Resonance Imaging

MRI is the dominant imaging modality in stroke because of the following:

1. MRI often reveals cerebral ischemia in its early stages, before it is visible on CT and often when the CT scan remains negative.

2. MRI frequently will reveal brainstem, cerebellar, or temporal lobe infarctions not visible on CT scan.

3. MRI is more accurate than CT in its ability to detect venous thrombosis as a cause of infarction.

4. MRI is more sensitive in detecting small infarctions (e.g., lacunes).

5. Diffusion-weighted MRI is the most sensitive technique in acute infarction. Echo-planar MRI is extraordinarily sensitive for hemorrhage and may replace CT in the future for this purpose.

6. Perfusion-weighted MRI may be useful for assessing the area of the brain "at-risk" for ischemia resulting from reduced perfusion.

7. MRA may be used as a screen for extracranial arterial stenosis, but it may overestimate the degree of stenosis. It is accurate in predicting total vessel occlusion and is helpful in assessing the posterior circulation (vertebrobasilar) system. It is not accurate in assessing intracranial arterial stenosis.

8. MRA and MRI in combination may show the location, size, and potentially the mechanism of stroke with one test. This combination of tests is most useful in thrombotic strokes, but may also be helpful in embolic strokes, lacunes, hemorrhages caused by AVM and berry aneurysm, and subarachnoid hemorrhage. Because of the duration of the study, uncooperative patients may be difficult to image without sedation or anesthesia. In addition, patients who are unstable may not be good candidates for such scanning. MRA may overestimate the degree of arterial stenosis and should be compared with another imaging modality.

9. CT remains preferable to MRI in the acute stroke patient when hemorrhage is a consideration and when patient cooperation is a problem. In addition, MRI is often not the first choice for patients with acute stroke because (a) patients are acutely ill and not as easily monitored as with CT, (b) CT is faster and more readily available, (c) CT is better in the patient with claustrophobia, and (d) CT is the benchmark study in assessing patients in acute stroke trials.

Noninvasive Vascular Testing

1. High-resolution color-flow duplex ultrasonography (DU) is a low-cost, risk-free, noninvasive technology that can provide useful information about the degree of carotid stenosis. In good laboratories, DU has achieved accuracy, sensitivity, and specificity of more than 90% when compared to percutaneous cut film cerebral angiography. Degree of stenosis generally is determined to be in categories of less than 20%, 20% to 39%, 40% to 59%, 60% to 79%, 80% to 99%, and 100% occlusion based on visual imaging information and Doppler spectral analysis of peak velocities of blood flow through the stenosis. When the visualization is good, DU

may also provide important information about plaque morphology (hemorrhage, cavitation, calcification, and stability), which may be important in determining the potential stroke risk. Because angiography is associated with a 1% to 2% risk of stroke or MI, many centers with validated laboratories have moved to using DU and MRA or CTa in concert to determine which patients may benefit from carotid endarterectomy.

2. TCD imaging allows assessment of the blood-flow characteristics of vessels in and about the circle of Willis. Because this region is not interrogated by DU, TCD is useful in assessing intracranial stenosis of the middle cerebral artery or vertebrobasilar system. TCD is technician dependent, and accuracy when compared to angiography may range from 60% to 85%. Still, when combined with MRA and when results are concordant, the test can be a quick and safe way to substantiate the clinical diagnosis of intracranial stenosis and guide the therapeutic approach. In addition, TCD is useful in assessing vasospasm in patients who have suffered subarachnoid hemorrhage from rupture of intracranial aneurysm. This largely has replaced angiography in the clinical setting because it is highly accurate (exceeding 90% sensitivity and specificity), is inexpensive, and can be done at the bedside at regular intervals to help guide the clinical management of these patients.

Arteriography

Arteriography, by conventional or digital method, is performed (a) to identify surgically correctable lesions (e.g., intracranial aneurysms and AVMs, carotid artery stenosis, and ulcerated carotid plaques), (b) to clarify an uncertain diagnosis, and (c) sometimes when anticoagulation is planned to be more certain of the diagnosis. In guiding arteriography, it is important to decide clinically whether disease is in the carotid or vertebrobasilar system. Wherever possible, arteriography should be done by selective catheterization techniques by an experienced radiologist. The cost and small but definite risk of stroke and other adverse reactions during arteriography must be weighed against the clinical value of the test in each patient.

CTa provides information about extracranial and intracranial vessels that may reduce the need for formal angiography. Intravenous dye is used for this study, with its attendant risks. CTa may be obtained rapidly and can be used as part of rapid stroke assessment.

Echocardiography

Echocardiography is useful in patients with a suspected cardiac source embolization. Transthoracic echocardiography has limited sensitivity to identify sources of embolism but may be positive with ventricular mural thrombi, large vegetations, valvular lesions, and congenital heart disease. "Bubble studies" may show right to left shunts, which potentiate paradoxic embolization. Transesophageal echocardiography often shows sources of embolism not visualized with transthoracic echo and is most helpful in young patients without obvious risk factors for stroke.

Lumbar Puncture

With the advent of CT scan, lumbar punctures are performed infrequently in the evaluation of the stroke patient. A lumbar puncture (see Chapter 30) is performed in the following situations:

- Meningitis is suspected.
- Subarachnoid hemorrhage is a diagnostic possibility. CT scans may be falsely negative in 5% to 10% of patients with subarachnoid hemorrhage. Subarachnoid hemorrhage shows grossly bloody CSF and usually an elevated CSF pressure.

TREATMENT

Risk factor modification and cholesterol-lowering regimens are key components of stroke treatment and even may reverse carotid stenosis (discussed later). Appropriate attention to smoking cessation, blood pressure, and diabetes control are crucial. HMG-CoA (3-hydroxy-3-methylglutaryl coenzyme A) reductase agents may reduce the risk of recurrent stroke by 30%, with or without hypercholesterolemia. There also has been recognition of the value of weight reduction, aerobic exercise, and proper diet in stroke prevention.

Cardiac Emboli—Anticoagulation

Anticoagulation

Anticoagulation is beneficial in preventing further embolization in patients with cardiac emboli (unless the source is bacterial endocarditis). Thus, diagnosing an embolus of cardiac origin is crucial. It is important to perform a CT scan or MRI to rule out bleeding before beginning anticoagulation. The timing of anti-coagulation after embolism remains controversial. Immediate anticoagulation therapy in patients with acute ischemic stroke is not associated with any short-term benefit (Gubitz et al., 2003). Recurrent embolus in the days after cardiac embolism occurs at a low rate, and the benefit of immediate anticoagulation seems to be counterbalanced by the risk of major bleeding. Particular caution and delay in anticoagulation are advised in elderly patients and in those with massive infarcts (greater than 5 cm in diameter) and uncontrolled hypertension. Begin with heparin, then switch to warfarin. An international normalization ratio (INR) of 2.0 to 3.0 appears to be required for effective stroke prevention in these patients. Higher levels of anticoagulation may be necessary for patients with metal prosthetic valves. If the embolus is caused by a mural thrombus associated with an MI, anticoagulation usually is continued for 6 months. Anticoagula-tion for 3 to 6 months sometimes is given for emboli of probable cardiac origin, although a definite cardiac source cannot be found. If atrial fibrillation or rheumatic valvular disease is the cause, long-term anticoagulation is indicated.

Carotid Stenosis

1. *Asymptomatic extracranial carotid stenosis*: In patients with severe stenosis, the risk of stroke is 2% per year with medical management alone. Less than 60% diameter stenosis is treated medically. In patients with more than 60% diameter stenosis, a large multicenter study (Asymptomatic Carotid Atherosclerosis Study, or ACAS) showed reduction of stroke from 2% to 1% per year in good-risk patients who under-went surgery. This favorable result depended on a surgical and angiographic morbidity and mortality of less than 3%.

2. *Symptomatic extracranial carotid stenosis*: The risk of stroke increases with increasing degrees of carotid stenosis. A large

multicenter study (North American Symptomatic Carotid Endarterectomy Trial, or NASCET) showed benefit of carotid surgery in medically stable patients with angiographically demonstrated 70% or greater diameter stenosis. Certain subgroups of symptomatic patients with moderate carotid stenosis (50% to 70%) benefit from surgery provided there is low surgical morbidity and mortality. Carotid angioplasty and stenting are being studied and may become an alternative to carotid endarterectomy, depending on complication rates.

3. *Completed carotid occlusion and stroke*: With completed carotid occlusion and stroke, urgent surgery appears to be of little benefit and may convert a bland infarction into a hemorrhagic one unless the surgery is performed within minutes of the stroke. Extracranial–intracranial vascular bypass has been found to be of no benefit in a large multicenter study. Similarly, short-term anticoagulation is used in many patients, but its value has not been proved in randomized studies.

Small-Vessel Lacunar Strokes

Antiplatelet therapy including aspirin, clopidogrel, or ASA/ dipyridamole usually is used to treat small-vessel lacunar strokes (see Chapter 16). In addition, risk factor modification is probably critical. There have been no major trials of therapy in patients with only small-vessel ischemic stroke.

General Care of Completed Infarction

1. Treatment in a specialized "stroke unit" is cost effective and improves outcome from stroke.
2. Urgent assessment of clinical status is imperative in thrombotic stroke. Newer agents are available that, in some cases, may change the course of the completed infarction.
3. In selected cases, tissue plasminogen activator (tPA) given intravenously according to a specific protocol appears to improve the functional outcome at 3 months in patients with moderate-sized infarctions of various mechanisms. In a multicenter trial, tPA appeared to be effective only when given in the first 3 hours after stroke. The hemorrhage rate in treated patients was 6.3% compared with placebo, in which the rate

was less than 1%. tPA should be administered only under the supervision of physicians experienced in its use in stroke and only when neurosurgical consultation is available.

4. Aspirin has been studied extensively for secondary prevention of stroke and reduces risk of nonfatal stroke, MI, and death by approximately 25% in most studies in patients with prior stroke or TIA. Clopidogrel (75 mg/day) and ASA/dipyridamole have slightly greater efficacy than aspirin in secondary stroke prevention.

5. Careful monitoring of the patient's status, attention to details of nursing such as prevention of deep vein thrombosis and decubiti, and prevention of aspiration from dysphagia are important in completed stroke.

6. Excessive blood pressure elevation should be treated cautiously. Moderate blood pressure elevation should not be treated because this may be a beneficial response to at-risk ischemic areas and often resolves on its own. Aggressive blood pressure treatment in the setting of acute infarction may cause a worsening of the stroke deficit because of further ischemia. Further studies are needed to assess the role of acute blood pressure management after ischemic stroke.

7. In patients with herniation, treatment with agents that reduce intracranial pressure may be helpful. Cranioplasty and duraplasty may be used as a rescue treatment for patients with major strokes who have massive life-threatening edema.

8. Cerebellar infarction with mass effect is a neurosurgical emergency. Immediate decompression may be life saving.

9. Heparinization should be avoided in large infarctions because of the risk of hemorrhage. Despite having been used in stroke therapy for years, heparin remains of unproven efficacy in the prevention of stroke or recurrent infarction.

Subarachnoid Hemorrhage, Subdural and Epidural Hemorrhage

Treatment of subarachnoid hemorrhage caused by aneurysm includes strict bed rest; control of blood pressure; and careful medical management including electrolyte monitoring, stool softeners, analgesia, and, whenever possible, early surgical clipping of the aneurysm. Without appropriate treatment, approximately 50% of those patients with subarachnoid hemorrhage who survive the first 24 hours will die within the next 2 weeks. The clinical condition of the patient, the presence of arterial spasm, and the location of the aneurysm influence surgical intervention. Vasospasm (narrowing of blood vessels on arteriography plus neurologic symptoms) usually begins 3 to 14 days after the initial bleed. Nimodipine, a calcium antagonist, reduces cerebral arterial vasospasm and usually is started immediately. There is a definite trend toward "early" aneurysm surgery after subarachnoid hemorrhage followed by volume expansion in an attempt to prevent rebleeding and to reduce vasospasm. Endovascular placement of coils in aneurysms has been shown to be superior to surgery in selected cases with small, accessible aneurysms.

Treatment of subdural and epidural hemorrhage is primarily neurosurgical but also depends on the chronicity of the bleeding, the size of the hemorrhage collection, and the status of the patient.

Intracerebral Hemorrhage

Treatment of increased intracranial pressure, stabilization of blood pressure, and consideration of neurosurgical decompression are important. Steroids have not been shown to be useful in the treatment of intracerebral hemorrhage. Nondominant putaminal hemorrhages or lobar hemorrhages with a risk of herniation may be helped by evacuation of the clot. Cerebellar hemorrhages with brainstem compression should be decompressed rapidly, if possible, to prevent irreversible brainstem injury. Massive intracerebral hemorrhages with brain injury are unlikely to be helped even with aggressive surgical treatment. Remember, identification of the cause of the hemorrhage and its mechanism (e.g., coagulopathy) is critical.

RECOVERY

Rehabilitation begins in the hospital as soon as possible and is best delivered as a comprehensive group of services tailored to the individual patient's needs. There is extensive literature supporting inpatient and outpatient rehabilitation in stroke patients. Functional recovery is improved by the early recognition and treatment of depression, which is common in stroke.

FUTURE

A variety of methods are being developed to lyse clot safely in the acute setting, decrease secondary brain injury from stroke, enhance cerebral recovery, and optimize diagnostic accuracy and safety. The particular type of stroke, its cause, and the associated medical condition of the patient are being considered in the treatment of stroke for the prevention of further stroke injury.

Suggested Reading

Adams HP, Adams RJ, Brott T, et al. Guidelines for the early management of patients with ischemic stroke. *Stroke* 2003;34:1056–1083.

Boiten J, Lodder J. Lacunar infarcts, pathogenesis and validity of the clinical syndromes. *Stroke* 1991;22:1374–1378.

Bougosslavsky J, Pierre P. Ischemic stroke in patients under age 45. *Neurol Clin* 1992;10:113–124.

Caplan LR. New strategies for stroke. *Arch Neurol* 1997;54:1222–1224.

Caprie Steering Committee. A randomized, blinded, trial of clopidogrel versus aspirin in patients at risk of ischemic events (CAPRIE). *Lancet* 1996;348:1329–1339.

Diener HC, Cunha L, Forbes C, et al. European Stroke Prevention Study 2. Dipyridamole and acetylsalicylic acid in the secondary prevention of stroke. *J Neurol Sci* 1996;143:1–13.

European Atrial Fibrillation Trial Study Group. *N Engl J Med* 1995;333:5–10.

Executive Committee of the Asymptomatic Carotid Atherosclerosis Study. Endarterectomy for asymptomatic carotid artery stenosis. *JAMA* 1995;273:1421–1428.

Gubitz G, Counsell C, Sandercock P, et al. Anticoagulants for acute ischaemic stoke (Cochrane Review). In: The Cochrane Library Issue 1 2003. Oxford: Update Software.

Kelley RE. Stroke prevention and intervention. New options for improved outcomes. *Postgrad Med* 1998;103:43–45.

Mohr JP, Thomas JC, Lazar RM, et al. A comparison of warfarin and aspirin for prevention of recurrent ischemic stroke. *N Engl J Med* 2001;345:1444–1451.

Molyneux A, Kerr R, Stratton I, et al. International subarachnoid aneurysm trial of neurosurgical clipping versus endovascular coils in 2143 patients with ruptured intracerebral aneurysms: a randomized trial. *Lancet* 2002;360:267–274.

Moore WS, Barnett HJ, Beebe HG, et al. Guidelines for carotid endarterectomy. A multidisciplinary consensus statement from the ad hoc committee, American Heart Association. *Stroke* 1995;26:188–201.

National Institute of Neurological Disorders and Stroke rt-PA Stroke Study Group. Tissue plasminogen activator for acute ischemic stroke. *N Engl J Med* 1995;333:1581–1587.

North American Symptomatic Carotid Endarterectomy Trial. Beneficial effect of carotid endarterectomy in symptomatic patients with high-grade carotid stenosis. *N Engl J Med* 1991;325:445–453.

Sacco RL. Risk factors, outcomes, and stroke subtypes for ischemic stroke. *Neurology* 1997;49:S39–S44.

Chapter 16

Selected Stroke Syndromes

Case

A 52-year-old woman comes to the emergency room with a headache and blood pressure of 220/130. She is weak in the left arm. Over the next 30 minutes, her speech becomes slurred, her left side becomes flaccid, she begins to have Cheyne-Stokes respirations, and she develops bilateral up-going toes. Her eyes and head are turned to the right.

Diagnosis

Right putaminal intracerebral hemorrhage, hypertensive.

LACUNES

Lacunes are vascular lesions in the brain commonly seen in patients with hypertension or diabetes. They are tiny areas of thrombotic infarction that become pea-sized holes pathologically. It is important to recognize lacunar strokes because they represent small-vessel disease and generally require limited investigation. Control of hypertension, hyperglycemia, and hyperlipidemia; cessation of smoking; and use of antiplatelet agents are likely to improve outcome and prevent future strokes. Look for these characteristic syndromes:

1. *Pure motor hemiplegia*: Lesion in the pons or internal capsule. Paralysis of face, arm, and leg without sensory loss. A right hemiplegia of lacunar origin has no accompanying aphasia; with a left hemiplegia, there are no parietal lobe findings.

2. *Pure sensory stroke*: Lesion most often in the thalamus. Sensory loss in face, arm, and leg, with no hemiplegia or other signs.
3. *Clumsy-hand dysarthria*: Lesion in the pons or internal capsule. Slurred speech with clumsiness and mild weakness of one arm.
4. *Crural (leg) paresis and ataxia (ataxic hemiparesis)*: Lesion in the pons or internal capsule. Ataxia and weakness of one leg.

Pure motor hemiplegia is the easiest to recognize; it occurs frequently.

INTRACEREBRAL HEMORRHAGE

Computed tomography (CT) scan is diagnostic in acute intracerebral hemorrhage.

Note: CT may miss hemorrhage in the brainstem and cerebellum because of bony artifacts. If the CT is "normal" and a clinical suspicion of posterior circulation hemorrhage remains, a magnetic resonance imaging scan should be obtained.

Bleeding into the cerebellum involves the following:

1. Cerebellar hemorrhage is important to diagnose because it can lead to rapid death via brainstem compression; treatment is surgical evacuation of the clot.
2. Headache, vomiting, and inability to walk with normal lower-extremity strength are cardinal features.
3. Strength and sensation are usually normal (unless brainstem compression occurs).
4. The patient may have trouble looking to the side of the lesion (gaze paresis).
5. Nystagmus and limb ataxia only occasionally are present.
6. Ipsilateral facial weakness may be present.
7. Cerebellar infarction with subsequent swelling may mimic cerebellar hemorrhage and require surgical treatment.

Most intracerebral hemorrhage occur in the *putamen*. Look for the following:

- Hemiplegia
- Striking eye deviation to side of hemorrhage and away from the hemiplegia (Fig. 16.1)
- Headache and often a field defect
- Cortical deficits, which develop as the hemorrhage progresses

Right putaminal hemorrhage

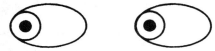

Eyes deviate to the side of the lesion.
Pupils: normal size and reactive.
(seen also with large hemisphere infarcts)

Thalamic hemorrhage

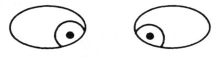

Eyes look down at the nose; vertical gaze is
impaired. Pupils: small and nonreactive.

Pontine hemorrhage

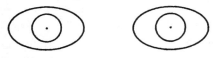

Eyes are midposition with no movement to doll's
eyes maneuver. There may be ocular bobbing.
Pupils: pinpoint, react to light if viewed with a
magnifying glass.

Cerebellar hemorrhage

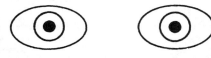

Patient has difficulty looking to the side of the
lesion. There may be skew deviation or a sixth
nerve palsy. Pupils: normal size and reactive.

FIGURE 16.1. Eye signs in intracerebral hemorrhage.

Surgical evacuation of the hematoma may be useful in nondominant hemisphere cases, particularly if the patient's condition deteriorates. Monitoring intracranial pressure is playing an increasing role in management. Control of blood pressure is important.

In *thalamic* hemorrhage, the patient displays the following characteristics:

- May or may not have hemiplegia
- Has eyes that look down at the nose, with small and nonreactive pupils (Fig. 16.1)
- Has marked sensory loss
- Supportive treatment is the only modality available.

Hemorrhage in the *pons* is usually fatal:

- The patient is comatose with small pinpoint pupils (Fig. 16.1).
- Pupils react to bright light when viewed with a magnifying glass.
- There is quadriparesis with up-going toes.
- Patient has no horizontal extraocular movements with passive head turning or use of ice water calorics.
- Ocular bobbing may occur (rapid downward eye deflection with slow upward drift).
- The patient may be locked in (conscious, but unable to move to show consciousness). He or she may retain the ability to look up and down.

Note: The most common causes of intracerebral hemorrhage are hypertension and trauma. Other causes include blood dyscrasias, side effects of anticoagulant therapy, drug abuse (cocaine), amyloid angiopathy, brain tumors, and cryptic arteriovenous malformations (AVMs).

SUBARACHNOID HEMORRHAGE

Subarachnoid hemorrhage (SAH) classically presents with the sudden onset of severe headache during activity, altered level of consciousness (at times coma), nuchal rigidity, and bloody cerebrospinal fluid. There may be autonomic disturbances such as vomiting, fever, and electrocardiogram changes. Up to 40% of patients with ruptured aneurysms experience a warning before the catastrophic bleeding. There are usually no focal signs, unless the hemorrhage is into the brain substance or arterial spasm exists. Hemorrhage into the brain substance appears as an increased density on CT scan; arterial spasm generally produces no changes on CT scan. Delayed deterioration in patients with SAH may be caused by hydrocephalus, seizures, cerebral edema, vasospasm, or rebleeding.

The most common locations for aneurysms are at various arterial junction points around the circle of Willis at the base of the brain:

1. Posterior communicating artery: may have associated third nerve palsy.
2. Anterior communicating artery: mutism and leg weakness may occur.
3. Middle cerebral artery: aphasia or nondominant hemisphere findings.
4. Less common locations include ophthalmic artery (unilateral blindness), cavernous sinus (ophthalmoplegia), and basilar artery (brainstem signs). AVMs may be found anywhere in the brain but are most common over the convexities. AVMs characteristically present with headaches, intracerebral hemorrhage, or SAH, with seizures.

Note: CT scan is abnormal in 90% of cases of SAH and has a false-negative rate of 10%. Therefore, do a lumbar puncture in suspected SAH when CT is "normal."

FOCAL THROMBOEMBOLIC STROKES

The *middle cerebral artery syndrome* seldom is caused by thrombosis of the middle cerebral artery; it is usually secondary to an occluded carotid in the neck or an embolus to the middle cerebral artery. Look for the following:

- Hemiparesis (greater in face and arm than in leg)
- Aphasia or nondominant hemisphere findings (depending on the side)
- Cortical sensory loss (greater in face and arm than in leg)
- Homonymous hemianopsia
- Conjugate eye deviation (to the side of the hemisphere lesion)

"Partial" middle cerebral artery syndromes, almost always of embolic origin, may include (a) sensorimotor paresis with little aphasia, (b) conduction aphasia, or (c) Wernicke's aphasia without hemiparesis.

In the anterior cerebral artery syndrome, look for the following:

- Paralysis of the lower extremity
- Cortical sensory loss in leg only
- Incontinence
- Grasp and suck reflexes
- Slowness in mentation with perseveration
- No hemianopsia or aphasia
- Limb apraxia

Occlusion of the *internal carotid artery* gives a picture resembling occlusion of the middle cerebral artery. When the anterior cerebral territory is included in the area of infarction, clinical features of anterior cerebral occlusion also occur. These patients tend to be stuporous or semicomatose because of the large area of infarction usually present.

The posterior cerebral artery syndrome presents these features:

- Homonymous hemianopsia (often the only finding); the patient may be unaware of the deficit
- Little or no paralysis
- Prominent sensory loss, including to pinprick and touch
- No aphasia or nondominant hemisphere dysfunction

Also, patients with left posterior cerebral artery syndrome may be unable to read but still may be able to write (alexia without agraphia) and to name colors. Recent memory loss may be present (involvement of hippocampus) or a confusional state initially.

Watershed or *border zone infarction syndromes* (common after anoxia) include proximal arm weakness with distal sparing and transcortical aphasia (see Chapter 4).

Brainstem syndromes never have cortical deficits or visual field defects. One of the most common brainstem syndromes is the *lateral medullary (Wallenberg's) syndrome* caused by occlusion of the vertebral or posterior inferior cerebellar artery (see Fig. 34.9). Look for the following:

- Ipsilateral to the lesion: facial numbness, limb ataxia, Horner's syndrome (miosis, ptosis, anhidrosis), pain over the eye

- Contralateral to the lesion: pinprick and temperature loss in arm and leg
- Vertigo, nausea, hiccups, hoarseness, difficulty swallowing, and diplopia

If the lesion is typical, treatment is supportive and these patients usually do well. (Beware of aspiration because of swallowing difficulty.)

Most other brainstem strokes are in the *pons* (see Fig. 34.8)

1. If the lesion is in the *medial* portion of the pons, there is weakness and an internuclear ophthalmoplegia or gaze palsy with little sensory loss.
2. If the lesion is in the *lateral and tegmental* portion of the pons, sensory loss predominates.
3. *Cerebellar* signs are present in lateral lesions and are ipsilateral to the lesion.
4. The *level* of the pons affected is determined by which cranial nerves are involved. The *facial* (seventh) nerve exits from the lower pons and, if involved there, produces ipsilateral total (upper and lower) facial paralysis. If involved higher, there is contralateral facial paralysis that spares the forehead musculature. The *trigeminal (fifth) nerve* exits from the middle of the pons and, if involved at this level, produces ipsilateral loss of corneal reflex and facial sensory loss. The descending tract of the trigeminal (nerve) runs from midpons to the upper cervical cord, and involvement anywhere in its course results in ipsilateral facial pinprick and temperature loss. In *high pontine* lesions, pain and sensory loss are contralateral to the lesion in the face and extremities. In brainstem lesions *below the high pons*, pain and temperature sensations are lost ipsilaterally in the face and contralaterally in the limbs. The cochlear (eighth) nucleus and nerve are in the lower pons; thus, ipsilateral deafness and vertigo may accompany pontine lesions.
5. Midbrain strokes frequently involve the third nerve or nucleus and cerebral peduncle, thus producing ipsilateral pupil dilatation, ptosis, ophthalmoparesis, and contralateral hemiplegia (Weber's syndrome) (see Fig. 34.7).

If the deficit in a brainstem stroke is confined to one anatomic area, it generally means that a single branch vessel is involved. If the deficit involves a wider area, the problem may be in the basilar artery and catastrophic basilar occlusion may result. Anticoagulation with heparin may prevent the progression from a partial to a complete basilar thrombosis.

Note: Rarely, stroke occurs in the spinal cord and presents as paraplegia with urinary retention; a sensory level usually can be found. Vibration and position sense are spared because the cause is often occlusion of the anterior spinal artery in patients with atherosclerotic disease with sparing of the posterior columns. The thoracic cord most often is affected. Treatment is symptomatic, and considerable recovery usually occurs.

Suggested Reading

Boiten J, Lodder J. Lacunar infarcts. *Stroke* 1991;22:1374–1378.

Feldmann E. Intracerebral hemorrhage. *Stroke* 1991;22:684–691.

Graff-Radford NR, Damasio H, Yamada T, et al. Nonhaemorrhagic thalamic infarction. *Brain* 1985;108:485–516.

Lehrich JR, Winkler GF, Ojemann RG. Cerebellar infarction with brainstem compression. *Arch Neurol* 1970;22:490–499.

Meyer FB, Morita A, Puumala MR, et al. Medical and surgical management of intracranial aneurysms. *Mayo Clin Proc* 1995;70:153–172.

Nader J, Bogousslavsky J. Natural history of patients with chronic occlusion of the internal carotid. *J Stroke Cerebrovasc Dis* 1993;3:202–207.

Chapter 17

Transient Ischemic Attack

The transient ischemic attack (TIA) is an acute neurologic deficit of vascular origin that clears completely; it usually lasts minutes to an hour, but by current definition remains no more than 24 hours. Recent data indicate that deficits lasting more than 30 minutes, even if symptoms resolve, are usually infarcts. TIAs are a symptom of disease, not a specific disorder. The mechanism of the TIA must be evaluated. Is it caused by large-vessel stenosis? Is it cardioembolic? Is there small vessel disease, which may present with TIA? Is there intracranial stenosis, such as in the basilar artery or middle cerebral artery? Symptoms of TIA are the same as symptoms of stroke, except for their transient nature. A TIA is important to recognize because it may be a warning that a more catastrophic and permanent neurologic deficit may be imminent. In some instances, treatment is available that will help prevent the impending stroke. Half to two thirds of people with thrombotic strokes give a history of a previous TIA, and approximately one fourth of patients with TIAs will have a stroke within 3 years. Many of these strokes occur within 2 days of the TIA. The following points should be established in the patient with a TIA.

IS THE TIA IN CAROTID OR VERTEBROBASILAR TERRITORY?

1. *TIAs in carotid distribution*: transient monocular blindness in the eye on the same side as a stenosed internal carotid artery (amaurosis fugax). The patient may report a "shade coming

down" over the eye or obscuration that appears like "white steam" over one eye.

- Transient aphasia
- Motor and sensory symptoms in a single extremity (upper or lower), involving face and arm (middle cerebral artery–territory involvement) or a clumsy ("bear's paw") hand.
- Motor and sensory deficits are similar in degree.

2. *TIAs in vertebrobasilar distribution*: slurred speech, dizziness, diplopia, ataxia, syncope, loss of consciousness, dysphagia, numbness around lips or face.

- Hemiparesis and hemisensory loss do not parallel each other in the individual limb as in carotid disease.
- There may be bilateral motor or sensory deficits from a single lesion.

3. *Lacunar or small-vessel thrombotic strokes*: occur abruptly or in a stuttering fashion over hours or days. There may be a warning; headache is absent, and hypertension or diabetes usually is present.

TIAs in *carotid territory* usually are associated with severe stenosis, but may be associated with moderate stenosis and ulcerative plaque at the carotid bifurcation in the neck. With carotid symptoms, especially in association with a carotid bruit or decreased carotid pulse, noninvasive carotid evaluation using carotid duplex ultrasound or magnetic resonance angiography (MRA) usually are performed to define the vascular anatomy and to determine whether the patient is a candidate for carotid endarterectomy. Computed tomography angiography also may be used for this determination. Occasionally, traditional cerebral arteriography may be necessary if the vascular anatomy is not well imaged with noninvasive techniques. Remember, the carotid must have a 75% cross-sectional area reduction before the blood flow is decreased significantly. If the TIA is caused by emboli from an ulcerated plaque, stenosis need not be present. There are patients who have an occluded internal carotid with no symptoms at all. Moreover, patients may have a carotid bruit without stenosis and stenosis without a bruit. There may be an occlusion with a palpable pulse or a decreased pulse in a patent vessel.

TIAs in the *vertebrobasilar territory*: the *vertebral arteries and their origins* have a predilection for atheroma development, and emboli of cardiac origin to the vertebrobasilar territory occur as do artery-to-artery embolism. Serious vertebrobasilar disease may be intracranial, in which surgery is not feasible, and the benefit of operation on the vertebral arteries in the neck is unproven.

In the *subclavian steal syndrome,* the patient has a narrowed subclavian artery proximal to the origin of the vertebral artery and the arm "steals" blood from the basilar artery through the vertebral artery. There may be a cervical bruit and a difference in blood pressure between arms. During exercise, the patient may experience symptoms of vertebrobasilar insufficiency. In contrast to other patients with TIAs, those with the subclavian steal syndrome rarely develop a stroke because of the steal, although there may be coexistent serious disease in the carotid arteries.

Vertigo alone is rarely a symptom of vertebrobasilar insufficiency unless other brainstem signs or symptoms are present. Occasionally, an elderly patient may have vertebrobasilar symptoms when turning the head, these being secondary to mechanical factors in the cervical region that reduce blood flow.

IS THE HEART THE SOURCE OF THE TIA?

Emboli from the heart are well-recognized causes of TIAs in the carotid and vertebrobasilar systems (more common in the carotid) and are seen in rheumatic heart disease, atrial fibrillation, mural thrombus after myocardial infarction, bacterial and marantic endocarditis, and atrial myxoma and with prosthetic valves. Cardiac emboli may cause TIAs, but they may be in different territories (e.g., first an episode of right-sided weakness, then an episode of left-sided weakness). Echocardiography is often helpful in diagnosis, especially in patients with known heart disease. Transesophageal echocardiography (TEE) is particularly helpful for detecting cardiac embolic sources such as mural thrombi or emboli from atherosclerosis in the ascending aorta. In addition, anomalies of the atria such as atrial septal aneurysm and atrial septal defect are imaged using TEE. Newer techniques, such as "bubble echocardiography," may detect small paradoxic emboli through a patent foramen ovale.

Cardiac arrhythmias may cause TIAs through decreased cardiac output and may require Holter monitoring for identification. Do not confuse Stokes-Adams attacks (syncope caused by heart block) with a TIA. Stokes-Adams attacks generally do not have focal neurologic symptoms or signs.

Hypotension may cause focal neurologic symptoms in a patient who has compromised cerebral circulation (e.g., as a result of stenosis of the internal carotid or middle cerebral artery).

IS THE "TIA" A MIGRAINOUS OR CONVULSIVE PHENOMENON?

Migraine may be accompanied by transient neurologic signs or symptoms (visual disturbances, motor or sensory) and usually can be identified by the headache that follows the neurologic deficit, by the gastrointestinal symptoms, and because it appears in patients younger than those with cerebrovascular disease. Nevertheless, older people experience migrainous phenomena, and there may not be prominent headache symptoms. Thus, migraine variants in the elderly post a difficult diagnostic and therapeutic problem. Migrainous sensory symptoms often "march" along an extremity ("marching numbness"). The time course of migraine aura is usually minutes, and there are usually some "positive symptoms" such as flashing lights, tingling, and the like.

Keep in mind that *focal seizures* may produce transient neurologic symptoms (numbness, leg or arm movement or weakness). The deficit is usually brief, lasting seconds unless there is focal status epilepticus. Obtain an electroencephalogram (EEG) if seizures are suspected. In addition, *chronic subdural hematoma* and *unruptured cerebral aneurysms* have been reported to present as recurrent transient neurologic deficits.

Some systemic factors may be associated with or may mimic TIAs. Such factors include anemia, polycythemia, thrombocytosis, and hyperglycemia and hypoglycemia. Hyperglycemia and hypoglycemia may unmask the expression of an old underlying neurologic deficit.

Transient global amnesia (TGA) is a unique syndrome in which, typically, a middle-aged patient suddenly loses recent memory, becomes confused, and asks the same questions repeatedly. The patient appears alert; has no motor or sensory signs or symptoms; and retains "personal identity" and the ability to answer questions about job, address, and so on. A characteristic feature is the repetition of the same questions by the patient despite being given the answer. The etiology of this dramatic syndrome is unknown, but theories include a migraine variant (favored), a seizure phenomenon, or ischemia involving the hippocampal system. Attacks of TGA often are triggered by special circumstances such as emotional experiences, pain, or sexual intercourse. Attacks usually last hours and clear without residual deficit. Unless attacks are recurrent, which is rare, treatment is usually unnecessary.

TREATMENT OF THE PATIENT WITH TIA

1. After a complete workup (including electrocardiogram, possibly Holter monitor or echocardiography, auscultation for bruits, blood pressure check in both arms, noninvasive tests such as Duplex ultrasound, MRA, and rarely EEG), arteriography may be necessary before deciding on a mode of treatment. Frequently, a combination of noninvasive vascular testing and MRA or cerebral tomographic angiography is replacing angiography in preoperative assessment for carotid endarterectomy. It is *critical* for the clinician to determine the cause of the transient neurologic deficit (e.g., embolism, migraine, arrhythmia) before embarking on a course of therapy.

2. Carotid endarterectomy is indicated when there is a unilateral severely stenosed (70% to 99% diameter) carotid in a patient with TIAs in that vessel's territory and if the surgery can be done with less than a 3% morbidity and mortality rate.

3. Some studies regarding *TIAs* have shown a statistically significant reduction of TIAs and subsequent strokes in patients treated with *anticoagulants*. However, most studies did not distinguish those patients with large- or small- vessel disease or those with TIAs in the anterior or posterior circulation, and arteriography was not carried out in all instances. Anticoagulation is indicated for patients with cardioembolic TIAs or where there is a coagulopathy causing TIA. Heparin often is used in patients with preocclusive stenosis after a TIA while awaiting surgery. There are no convincing data to support this practice. For those who have an ulcerated or irregular plaque without severe stenosis that may form the nidus of embolic material, or in those with small-vessel disease,

antiplatelet agents are used (e.g., aspirin, ASA/disopyramide, or clopidogrel). There is no evidence that anticoagulation benefits patients with small-vessel disease, a completed stroke, or a completely occluded large vessel.

4. We still favor the following guidelines for the management of TIAs (assuming that mimickers of TIA, such as migraine and seizures, have been excluded)

   ■ Most patients with vertebrobasilar TIAs are treated medically.

   ■ If a skilled surgeon is available, patients with typical carotid TIAs who are suitable medical risks should have carotid endarterectomy if an appropriate lesion (e.g., greater than 70% diameter stenosis) is found. Patients with a 50% to 70% symptomatic carotid lesion (moderate) benefit from surgery, although less so than those with more stenotic lesions.

   ■ Patients with TIAs caused by large-vessel occlusive disease of less than 2 months' duration who do not receive surgery are treated with 3 months of warfarin therapy (unless contraindicated) before treatment with aspirin, ASA/dipyridamole, or clopidogrel is begun. Data from the Warfarin versus Aspirin in Recurrent Stroke study (WARSS) did not indicate a benefit of Coumadin over aspirin for patients with large-vessel stenotic lesions (see Mohr et al., 2001).

   ■ Patients with continuing TIAs of 2 or more months' duration who do not receive surgery are treated with antiplatelet agents unless there has been a recent increase in the frequency, duration, or severity of TIAs. Under these circumstances, warfarin therapy is advised for 3 months before aspirin is started. Antiplatelet therapy should be continued indefinitely.

A patient is more likely to have a stroke after a few recent TIAs than after TIAs occurring in the distant past. There are a large number of TIAs for which no etiology (i.e., 40% cryptogenic) can be found (e.g., normal cerebral arteriogram and normal cardiac status); this obviously makes the rationale for treatment difficult. Possible explanations include the following:

■ Some TIAs may be associated with small-vessel disease not demonstrable on angiography.

- Emboli that result in TIAs may break up as the TIA resolves.
- Patients with TIAs and a negative workup usually are treated with aspirin, ASA/dipyridamole, or clopidogrel.

Suggested Reading

Hodges JR. Unraveling the enigma of transient global amnesia. *Ann Neurol* 1998;43:151–153.

Humphrey PR. Management of transient ischaemic attacks and stroke. *Postgrad Med J* 1995;71:577–584.

Mohr JP, Thomas JC, Lazar RM, et al. A comparison of warfarin and aspirin for prevention of recurrent ischemic stroke. *N Engl J Med* 2001;345:1444–1451.

Moore WS, Barnett HJ, Beebe HG, et al. Guidelines for carotid endarterectomy. A multidisciplinary consensus statement from the ad hoc committee, American Heart Association. *Stroke* 1995;26:188–201.

North American Symptomatic Carotid Endarterectomy Trial. Beneficial effect of carotid endarterectomy in symptomatic patients with high-grade carotid stenosis. *N Engl J Med* 1991;325:445–453.

Welsh JE, Tyson GW, Winn HR, et al. Chronic subdural hematoma presenting as transient neurologic deficits. *Stroke* 1979;10:564.

Chapter 18

Headache

Case

A 32-year-old right-handed accountant began having headaches twice a month at age 15. She remembers her mother going to bed in a dark room with "sinus" headaches. The patient's headaches are severe, pounding, and unilateral; located in the right or left temple; and associated with nausea and photophobia. Some headaches are preceded by zigzag, colored lights. Red wine predictably brings on her headaches. Treatment with beta blockers makes her headaches less frequent. The acute headaches usually are relieved with naproxen sodium. For more severe headaches, she uses an oral triptan.

Diagnosis

Migraine with and without visual aura.

Critical to the evaluation of the patient with headache is obtaining a careful history. It is important to distinguish the three major types of "benign" headache (migraine, cluster, and tension-type headache) and recognize the warning signs of the more ominous headache. Features that provide crucial information include the character of the headache, its timing and duration, exacerbating and relieving factors, and associated symptoms.

CHARACTER OF THE HEADACHE PAIN

Migraine headaches are periodic, throbbing headaches; usually unilateral; and over one eye or in the temple. Photophobia and sensitivity to sound are common, as are nausea and vomiting. Scalp sensitivity is also common. Associated symptoms may precede the headache (migraine with aura), or the headache may occur alone (migraine without aura). There is frequently a family history of migraine and childhood motion sickness, and symptoms often begin during teenage years. Migraine is more common in females.

Cluster headaches are sharp, knifelike, and unilateral and often are over one eye. They are more common in males and begin later in life than do migraine headaches.

Tension-type headaches tend to be diffuse, steady, nonthrobbing headaches in the front or back of the head. They are bilateral and often described as "bandlike" or "tight" headaches. They occur in all age groups.

TIMING AND DURATION

Migraine headaches are periodic, lasting a few hours to a few days. They may occur at any time and may awaken the patient from sleep. They often begin during a "relaxed" time (e.g., the weekend). Status migrainosus refers to migraine that lasts for days.

Cluster headaches come in groups over a few weeks or months (a cluster) and then subside. They last for a few minutes to 1 to 2 hours and tend to occur at the same time every day. They may awaken a patient 1 or 2 hours after falling asleep.

Tension-type headaches usually last hours but may last days, weeks, and even months. They frequently occur at the end of a stressful day.

EXACERBATING AND RELIEVING FACTORS

Migraine may be exacerbated or relieved during menstruation or pregnancy or at the time of menopause. Migraine often is relieved by sleep or after vomiting. Migraine may be brought on by hunger; alcohol ingestion; caffeine withdrawal; and certain foods such as aged cheese, cured meats, and chocolate. The use of birth control pills often worsens migraine.

Cluster headaches often are precipitated by alcohol, sometimes exquisitely so. Cluster headaches usually are not relieved by environmental factors until they have run their course.

Tension-type headaches may be relieved with relaxation, neck massage, or rest.

ASSOCIATED SYMPTOMS

Migraine with aura may be accompanied by a variety of neurologic symptoms, often immediately preceding the headache. These include such visual symptoms as flashing lights, zigzag lines, blind spots, or complete loss of a visual field. These last for minutes, and the headache usually begins as the visual symptoms recede. Other symptoms that occur are characterized by a gradual change over minutes from one symptom to another, such as hemianopsia to difficulty talking, tingling of one hand to tingling of the entire side, or progression to actual hemiparesis ("hemiplegic migraine"). Confusion, vertigo, stupor, and ataxia are less common manifestations of migraine. Sometimes "positive symptoms" such as flashing lights are followed by "negative" ones such as visual loss.

In *cluster* headaches, tearing, facial flushing, and a stuffy, runny nose are common, and usually ipsilateral to the headache. Sometimes Horner's syndrome may accompany the headache (small pupil, ptosis).

Tension-type headache tends to be isolated without associated symptoms.

HEADACHE AND DEPRESSION

Depression may present with headache, and chronic headache patients frequently have depression as part of their symptom complex. Exploring issues such as new stress at home or work, domestic strife, illness at home, or recent bereavement may be key in understanding a new or changed headache. Assessment of depression is an important part of chronic headache assessment, although one must be careful before ascribing the headache to depression alone.

OMINOUS HEADACHES

Occasionally, a patient presenting with a new or changed headache is harboring a major illness that requires diagnosis and treatment. The following symptoms are suggestive of an ominous cause and, if present, require careful evaluation:

1. A change in character, pattern, or timing of a preexisting headache
2. A new-onset headache
3. Headache associated with persistent neurologic signs or symptoms
4. A sudden, severe "worst headache of my life" (subarachnoid hemorrhage)
5. A progressive headache over days or weeks (mass lesion)
6. Stiff neck, fever, altered mental status (meningitis or encephalitis)
7. Headache with jaw pain, systemic symptoms, visual blurring (temporal arteritis)

EXAMINATION OF THE PATIENT WITH HEADACHE

Examination sometimes offers clues to the type of headache or to the presence of organic causes, especially if the patient is symptomatic during the examination.

1. Look carefully for *focal signs* suggesting a tumor or other structural lesions. (Make sure to check the fundi for papilledema.)
2. Check for *autonomic dysfunction* during headache for cluster (e.g., miotic pupil, ptosis, red eye, tearing, unilateral nasal congestion).
3. Note "sweaty" hands and feet and scalp tenderness (migraine).
4. Check for *meningismus* (subarachnoid hemorrhage, meningitis).
5. Listen for *bruit* over one eye, skull, and neck (arteriovenous malformation, carotid-cavernous fistula, severe carotid stenosis).
6. Headache over the eye in a person older than 50 may be caused by *temporal arteritis.* Check for a tender temporal artery or nodularity of the artery.
7. Note hypertension, which may exacerbate migraine or tension headaches, particularly if the hypertension is labile.
8. Glaucoma is a cause of headache in the elderly; headache, eye pain, red eye, and vomiting are common. Palpate the

globe, and perform tonometry if glaucoma is suspected. Treatment with medication or eye surgery may prevent blindness; thus, early diagnosis is crucial.

9. Constant headache in an obese female may be caused by pseudotumor cerebri. It is associated with papilledema as a result of increased intracranial pressure (see Chapter 30).

10. Occipital headache may be caused by cervical arthritis, especially in the elderly. Exacerbation of pain by neck movement is helpful in the diagnosis.

Note: Temporal arteritis and glaucoma may present as headache in the elderly, and either may lead to blindness.

LABORATORY STUDIES

Laboratory studies in the patient with headache depend on the clinical impression after obtaining the history and performing a careful examination. All headache sufferers probably should receive a complete blood count, chemistry screen, and sedimentation rate. Beyond that, individualize.

1. If the history suggests tension headache and the examination is normal, a treatment trial without further testing is reasonable.

2. Most patients with common or classic migraine deserve a computed tomography (CT) scan or magnetic resonance imaging (MRI) at least once for reassurance that another process (e.g., arteriovenous malformation, infarcts caused by migraine) is not being overlooked.

3. CT or MRI is mandatory for a patient with ominous headache symptoms or if there is a focal neurologic deficit or signs of increased intracranial pressure.

4. Electroencephalogram is no longer helpful in headache assessment except in the case of patients suspected of harboring concurrent seizure activity, which may respond to antiepileptic medication.

5. Additional specific studies are used depending on the circumstances (e.g., serum lead level in a car mechanic or arterial blood gases in a patient with chronic lung disease suspected of CO_2 narcosis).

TREATMENT TIPS

Headache therapy first consists of altering environmental factors. Tapering off caffeinated beverages, avoiding precipitating foods and drink, getting regular exercise, altering changeable stressors, and performing relaxation exercises all have a place in therapy. Some patients develop a refractory headache disorder (transformed headache) caused by the regular use of headache medications and must be "detoxified" before treatment can be effective.

Migraine

Treatment of Acute Headache

1. *Aspirin or acetaminophen* may help but usually have been tried already.
2. *Caffeine* in combination with aspirin or acetaminophen is often useful.
3. Therapy with *nonsteroidal analgesics* (naproxen sodium, ibuprofen, tolfenamic acid) may be effective.
4. The *triptans* are serotonin receptor agonists that act by constricting cranial vessels and by inhibiting chemical mediators in peripheral branches of the trigeminal nerve. They vary in route of administration, time to maximum effect, duration of effect, and side effect profile.
   - *Sumatriptan* is a 5-hydroxytryptamine receptor agonist available in injection, nasal spray, and pill form and is effective in acute migraine.
   - *Zolmitriptan* is a serotonin agonist for acute headache therapy available only in pill form.
   - Other available triptans include almotriptan, eletriptan, frovatriptan, naratriptan, rizatriptan, and zolmitriptan.
   - One should become familiar with two or three of the triptan medicines to understand their efficacy and learn their side effect profiles.
5. *Fiorinal,* although effective, often leads to an overuse syndrome. It should be used with caution.
6. *Antinauseants,* such as chlorpromazine, may be helpful for nausea and headache. They may improve gastrointestinal motility and facilitate absorption of more specific antimigraine medications.

7. *Ergot* derivatives in various forms are useful. Intranasal dihydroergotamine may be effective. Ergot derivatives are contraindicated in hemiplegic migraine and in patients with known coronary vasospasm or peripheral vascular disease.

8. A *stratified care* model often is used, in which the patient takes different medications depending on the severity of the headache. This reduces treatment failures and ensures that appropriate medication is used early in the headache when it is most likely to be effective.

9. Combination therapy may be more effective than individual agents alone.

10. Narcotics are seldom necessary.

11. Remember, emphasize prevention over acute treatment.

Prophylactic Medication

1. *Tricyclic antidepressants (TCAs),* such as amitriptyline and nortriptyline, are useful in migraine prophylaxis, especially with coexisting depression and tension-type headaches. Selective serotonin reuptake inhibitors are not as effective as TCAs in migraine prophylaxis.

2. The *antiepileptic medication* valproic acid is effective in migraine prophylaxis, although careful monitoring for idiosyncratic reactions is important. Other antiepileptic medications that may be used in migraine prophylaxis include topiramate, lamotrigine, and gabapentin.

3. Beta blockers are an effective class of medications for migraine prophylaxis, with propranolol, atenolol, and nadolol being most effective. Long-acting preparations are available. Some patients respond to a second beta blocker after not responding to the first. Contraindications include asthma, diabetes, heart failure, heart block, depression, pregnancy, and Raynaud's phenomenon.

4. *Calcium-channel blockers* are less useful than initially thought, and results of trials of their use are disappointing. They may be worthwhile in patients with a prolonged aura or coexisting Raynaud's or Prinzmetal's angina and in hemiplegic migraine.

5. Nonsteroidal medications (e.g., naproxen sodium) or estrogen supplementation may be particularly helpful in menstrual migraine therapy.

Cluster Headaches

1. Cluster headaches may be refractory to treatment once headache is established.
2. Oxygen via a non-rebreather mask at a flow rate of 7 liters for 15 minutes provides relief in approximately 70% of patients.
3. Subcutaneous sumatriptan is very effective for the acute treatment of cluster headache. There does not appear to be tachyphylaxis with daily use in cluster headache. It is not useful as a prophylactic medicine.
4. Dihydroergotamine (DHE) in intravenous form is effective in cluster headache but usually cannot be given in time by that route. Intranasal DHE is less effective but helps some patients.
5. Zolmitriptan in 5- to 10-mg oral doses is effective in cluster headaches, although less so than subcutaneous sumatriptan.
6. Intranasal lidocaine 4% spray has a modest effect and may be used in an adjunctive capacity in cluster headache.
7. Transitional prophylaxis during a cluster may be used to bridge to a more long-term prophylactic agent. Oral ergotamine tartrate 2 mg or DHE 1 mg intramuscularly can be used daily during a cluster with effective prevention of headaches. Both are contraindicated in patients with vascular disease or uncontrolled hypertension or during pregnancy. A short course of steroids may be effective in transitional prophylaxis.
8. Maintenance prophylaxis is used for the expected duration of the cluster period. The following medications have shown efficacy in randomized placebo-controlled trials: verapamil, lithium carbonate, methysergide, valproic acid, and topiramate. Each medication has its own set of side effects, which should be reviewed with the patient.
9. In chronic cluster headache, indomethacin and lithium may be effective.

Tension Headache

1. Aspirin, acetaminophen, and nonsteroidal antiinflammatory drugs commonly are used.
2. Recurrent tension-type headaches may respond to lifestyle changes. Remember, some medications or medical condi-

tions (e.g., chronic renal failure) may make tension headache worse.

3. Make sure the patient does not have a medication overuse headache (see later in this chapter).
4. TCAs may be helpful in the prevention of chronic tension-type headaches.
5. Neck massage, cervical pillow, relaxation exercises, and nontraditional therapies (e.g., acupuncture) may be helpful.
6. Regular physical exercise is helpful in most patients.

Headache Associated with Depression

Antidepressants may relieve headache in certain instances. Psychotherapy may be necessary.

Medication Overuse Headache

Patients who frequently use analgesics, narcotics, caffeine, or the triptan medications may develop medication overuse headache or a "transformed" headache. The overuse causes drug-rebound headaches, leading to even more dependence on medication in a vicious cycle. In European headache centers, up to 10% of patients have this headache type. There are no specific guidelines for "how much is too much" medication. As a general rule, three or more acute headache medications for 5 days a week is excessive, with even less frequent dosing recommended for triptans and opiates. Many patients develop a progressively increasing attack frequency, with a reduction in headache-free periods. The character of the headaches may change to a more constant, tension-type headache pattern. The frequent use of headache medication interferes with the efficacy of prophylactic medications, and patients often report failing multiple preventive drugs. It is crucial to educate the patient about the syndrome and develop a strategy for withdrawing the offending medications or drugs. This may be done in either an outpatient or inpatient setting. Once patients are no longer taking the acute medications, the headache character may revert to its original periodic pattern and respond to standard preventive therapies.

Suggested Reading

Capobianco DJ, Cheshire WP, Campbell JK. An overview of the diagnosis and pharmacologic treatment of migraine. *Mayo Clin Proc* 1996;71: 1055–1066.

Edmeads J. The worst headache ever: ominous and inominous causes. *Postgrad Med* 1989;86:93–104, 107–110.

Ferrera PC, Reicho PR. Acute confusional migraine and trauma-triggered migraine. *Am J Emerg Med* 1996;14:276–278.

Headache Classification Committee of the International Headache Society. Classification and diagnostic criteria for headache disorders, cranial neuralgias and facial pain. *Cephalalgia* 1988;8(Suppl 7):1–96.

Lipton, RB, Scher AL, Kolodner K. Migraine in the United States: epidemiology and patterns of health care use. *Neurology* 2002;58: 885–894.

Mathew NT, Kurman R, Perez F. Drug induced refractory headache—clinical features and management. *Headache* 1990;30:634–638.

Silberstein SD. Evaluation and emergency treatment of headache. *Headache* 1992;32:396–407.

Silberstein SD. Tension-type and chronic daily headache. *Neurology* 1993;43:1644–1649.

Silberstein SD, Merriam GR. Estrogens, progestins, and headache. *Neurology* 1991:41:786–793.

Silverman K, Evans SM, Strain EC, et al. Withdrawal syndrome after the double-blind cessation of caffeine consumption. *N Engl J Med* 1992: 327:1109–1114.

Spierings EL. Mechanism of migraine and action of antimigraine medications. *Med Clin North Am* 2001;85:943–958.

US Headache Consortium. Guidelines for headache management. www.ahsnet.org/guidelines.php.

Von Seggern RL, Adelman JU. Cost considerations in headache treatment, part 2: acute migraine treatment. *Headache* 1996;36:493–502.

Weingarten S, Kleinman M, Elperin L, et al. The effectiveness of cerebral imaging in the diagnosis of chronic headache. *Arch Intern Med* 1992: 152:2457–2462.

Welch KMA. Drug therapy of migraine. *N Engl J Med* 1993;329: 1476–1483.

Chapter 19

Dementia

Case

An 82-year-old retired schoolteacher has had increasing problems functioning at home. She stopped driving a year ago after she became lost on the way home from church. Nine months ago, her daughter took over paying the bills and grocery shopping when she realized her mother could no longer balance her checkbook or make a shopping list. Five months ago she began to misidentify her son as her deceased husband, and 3 months ago she began to have trouble reading the newspaper and getting dressed. She repeats herself frequently, and she leaves the stove on after cooking. In the past month, she has been hiding her jewelry around the house for fear it might be stolen. Her neurologic examination is unremarkable except for a mini-mental status examination score of 16 out of a possible score of 30.

Diagnosis

Probable senile dementia of the Alzheimer type.

Dementia is a loss of intellectual ability that interferes with a person's ability to function at work or in a social situation. There are many causes of dementia, the most common being Alzheimer's disease (AD) and multi-infarct dementia (MID). Treatments for AD have become available, increasing the importance of establishing a diagnosis. The goal of the physician is to characterize the patient's dementia, to search for a treatable cause and appropriate therapy, and to provide the patient and family with practical information for coping with the illness.

WHAT IS THE NATURE OF THE DEMENTIA?

Obtain a Careful History

1. A careful history from the family is essential. Never depend on the patient's account alone.
2. When did problems first begin and how rapidly have they progressed? Include questions about working, driving, shopping, doing the checkbook, and self-grooming.
3. Is there a problem with language? Does the patient have trouble finding words, or does the patient use unusual words (paraphasic errors)? These suggest a dominant-hemisphere language area abnormality.
4. Is there a change in personality (i.e., more irritable or more placid)? Such changes may be seen in frontal lobe dementias, as well as in later stages of AD.
5. Has the patient lost initiative (e.g., given up hobbies or suggesting where to go on weekends)? This is seen particularly with frontal lobe disorders.
6. Does the patient get lost in the house or lose the car in a parking lot? This may suggest nondominant parietal dysfunction.
7. Is the patient ataxic or incontinent? Normal pressure hydrocephalus (NPH) causes the triad of dementia, ataxia, and incontinence.
8. Is there evidence of depression? In the elderly, depression may mimic dementia and respond to antidepressants.
9. Are there medications, toxins, or "sleeping pills" that could be compromising intellect? Substance abuse (e.g., alcohol) and medication toxicity frequently are underdiagnosed in the elderly.
10. Are there medical illnesses that may have an impact on cognition? Is the patient positive for the human immunodeficiency virus (HIV), which is a major cause of dementia in younger adults?
11. Is there a family history of dementia? Often, this may be covered up by the family. Ask about "senility" or failing faculties in the elderly.

12. Is there a history of stroke, hypertension, diabetes, or other vascular risk factors? These may point to MID.

13. Are there concurrent parkinsonism, mental fluctuations, and formed visual hallucinations? Lewy body dementia has these features.

14. Is there progressive headache or focal neurologic symptoms to suggest a mass lesion?

Define the Mental Status

There are readily available brief mental status tests (e.g., Folstein mini-mental status, short test of mental status) that can be used as screening tools and are quantitative. Thus, they can be used to objectively observe patients. Definition of the mental status consists of the following components:

1. *State of consciousness.* If the patient is not fully awake, one should suspect a metabolic disorder or a space-occupying lesion. Clues that the process may be *delirium* rather than dementia include inattention, fluctuating symptoms, disturbances in sleep, prominent perceptual abnormalities, and increased autonomic activity.

2. *Orientation* to place, person, and time. Also check for attention by digit span or by having patient recite months of the year backwards. If a patient is inattentive, it is difficult to interpret the rest of the mental status examination.

3. *Aphasia* (see Chapter 4). Test ability to read a newspaper and write to dictation. If so, were there errors?

4. *New memory.* Can the patient recall three or four unrelated objects after 5 minutes? Can the patient remember money placed under the pillow or in a pajama pocket? Test knowledge of recent current events.

5. *Old memory.* Can the patient give correct information about events that occurred some years ago (e.g., naming of presidents)?

6. *Calculation.* Give a simple problem, such as "four rolls cost 24 cents each" or "if you give the baker $1.00, how much change would you receive?"

7. *Abstraction.* Ask questions such as "How are a ball and an orange alike?" or "What do a bathtub and the ocean have in common?"

8. *Judgment.* What would the patient do in situations such as spotting a fire in a theater or finding a stamped, addressed envelope in the street?
9. *Pictures.* How well can the patient interpret a picture in a magazine? Is there focus on one tiny part and an inability to integrate it (visual agnosia)? Can the patient draw or copy designs (constructional apraxia)?
10. *Mood and thought content.* Is the patient sad or inappropriately cheerful? Fearful or paranoid? Active or apathetic? Personally neat or sloppy? Is the patient's affect labile?

Perform Careful General and Neurologic Examinations

1. For the general examination, is there evidence of liver, kidney, lung, heart, adrenal, or thyroid disease?
2. Is the blood pressure elevated? Is the heart rhythm regular?
3. Are there focal neurologic signs, papilledema, or nonspecific signs of cerebral dysfunction such as grasp responses, snout, or palmomental reflex? Are the reflexes brisk? Are the toes up-going?
4. Check vision and hearing. Symptoms of dementia are made worse by sensory deprivation. Test for smell.
5. Is the gait abnormal? Are there signs of parkinsonism?

DO THE HISTORY AND PHYSICAL SUGGEST A TREATABLE CAUSE?

Although treatable causes of a dementia are not common, it is important to screen for the known treatable causes of dementia because, if found, treatment can significantly improve or reverse abnormal mental function.

Is There a Tumor?

1. Tumors presenting silently as dementia are often in the frontal lobe. Frontal lobe reflexes (suck, snout, grasp) may be present, and there is a "slowness" in carrying out tasks. Smell may be impaired. Tumors occurring in other areas usually give focal signs. Seizures and gait disorders are common features of brain tumors.
2. Tumors obstructing the third or fourth ventricle may cause hydrocephalus and subsequent dementia, often with few

focal signs. Intermittent exacerbation of symptoms is common because of transient obstruction of the cerebrospinal fluid (CSF) pathway.

3. Memory difficulties or language problems are not common early features of brain tumors.

4. The patient with dementia secondary to brain tumor usually presents clear evidence of the tumor within 6 to 12 months of the onset of dementia (see Chapter 23 for signs and symptoms of brain tumor.)

5. A normal computed tomography (CT) scan, with and without contrast, is usually sufficient to rule out tumor. Magnetic resonance imaging (MRI) is more sensitive than CT scan for brain tumor, especially for those located in the posterior fossa.

Normal Pressure Hydrocephalus

1. Consider NPH when mental deterioration occurs over 6 to 12 months and there is an associated gait disorder and incontinence. Up-going toes are common.

2. The pathophysiology of NPH is not well understood, but it involves inadequate absorption of CSF over the cerebral hemispheres, leading to hydrocephalus.

3. NPH may follow subarachnoid hemorrhage, meningitis, or head trauma, but it is often of unknown etiology.

4. No test is specific or diagnostic of NPH, although large ventricles in the absence of cortical atrophy are highly suggestive.

5. Improvement in gait after lumbar puncture (LP) and removal of CSF may be a helpful clue to the diagnosis.

6. If NPH is a serious consideration, MRI is indicated. The patients who are most likely to benefit from a shunt procedure are those with a "characteristic" clinical history and a short period of deterioration and those who have gait disorder and incontinence as the initial symptoms.

7. Complications after shunting are common and include aspiration, infection, and subdural hematoma.

Chronic Subdural Hematoma

Sometimes after minor trauma or trauma that is not remembered by the patient, slowly progressive subdural hematomas present with dementia. Headache, fluctuating symptoms, a gait abnormality, and relatively short-term progression are suggestive. Sometimes an isodense subdural will be missed on CT, so consider MRI. Do not perform an LP because it is not diagnostic and may cause herniation.

B$_{12}$ Deficiency

Altered cognitive function is becoming better recognized as a consequence of B$_{12}$ deficiency. Onset may be insidious over months or years. Patients may not have the usual hematologic changes before neurologic symptoms. A borderline B$_{12}$ may be significant, and other confirmatory testing such as homocysteine level and methylmalonic acid level usually will be elevated if there is a true deficiency. Antiparietal cell antibodies or intrinsic factor antibodies are usually positive in pernicious anemia. The Schilling test may be negative in patients with primarily neurologic symptoms of B$_{12}$ deficiency. Look for associated paresthesias and posterior and lateral column spinal cord signs (combined system disease; see Chapter 13).

Metabolic Diseases

Patient with dementia secondary to hepatic, renal, and endocrine diseases usually do not have a clear sensorium. In young patients with liver disease and dementia or depression, check for Wilson's disease (ceruloplasmin and 24-hour urinary copper). Check for hypothyroidism, and consider the possibility of hypoglycemia (e.g., in a patient with diabetes being treated with insulin) and Cushing's disease.

Infectious Diseases

Consider CSF examination in selected patients for tuberculosis or fungal or carcinomatous meningitis. Patients with acquired immunodeficiency syndrome (AIDS) may develop an encephalopathy with behavioral changes and dementia (HIV-associated dementia). Syphilis serology is no longer routinely obtained unless: (a) the patient is at high risk (e.g., AIDS); (b) there are signs or symptoms suggesting syphilis; or (c) the patient lives in an endemic area for syphilis.

Drug and Toxins

Sleeping medication, antianxiety drugs, and alcohol are important causes of cognitive dysfunction in the elderly. Barbiturates and benzodiazepines may cause cognitive dysfunction. Patients may not consider sleeping pills to be "medication" and may not list them on forms.

Depression

Depression may present as dementia in the elderly, and this condition sometimes is referred to as a "pseudodementia." Suggestive features include a history of psychiatric disease; a relatively brief duration of symptoms; and vegetative symptoms of depression, including anorexia, weight loss, altered sleep pattern, decreased concentration, loss of energy, and psychomotor retardation. Specific features of depression include sadness, guilt, apathy, social withdrawal, episodes of weeping, and suicidal ideas. Pseudodementia has been shown to presage true dementia in some patients; therefore, treatment of the depression may be only part of the required therapy.

Other Treatable Causes

Rarer causes of treatable dementia include thiamine deficiency, carbon monoxide poisoning, congestive heart failure, chronic hypoxia, untreated hypertension, hypercalcemia, carcinoma of the lung, subacute bacterial endocarditis, and porphyria. All may include dementia in their clinical picture.

ALZHEIMER'S DISEASE AND OTHER DEMENTIAS

Alzheimer's Disease

The most common cause of dementia is AD. Onset before age 65 years and after age 65 was once thought to be different diseases, but now is recognized to represent a spectrum of onset of a common pathology. The following features are characteristic of the disease:

1. Progression is slow, over years, without stepwise change.
2. Gradually developing forgetfulness is the key feature, eventually accompanied by problems with other cognitive tasks.

Day-to-day events, names, places, and directions to familiar sites all may be forgotten. Language problems with difficulty finding certain words may occur. Problems with mathematics are common, usually manifested with using the checkbook. Visuospatial problems occur (e.g., analyzing a picture, difficulty drawing or copying figures, or difficulty figuring out how mechanical appliances work). Alertness is preserved until late stages.

3. The patient often is brought to the physician by the family and is unaware that there is a problem.

4. There are usually no neurologic signs apart from the dementia; toes are usually down-going, and the patient is generally sociable and neat in the early stages. A grasp or snout response may be present. Later, personality change is frequent. There sometimes is visual agnosia (the ability to see parts of, but not recognize, objects) and motor apraxia (inability to perform certain stereotyped motor tasks in the absence of paralysis). At advanced stages, seizures may occur infrequently.

5. A substantial subset of patients with AD develops extrapyramidal signs late in the disease.

6. CT or MRI shows nonspecific findings of atrophy and ventricular dilatation. Electroencephalogram (EEG) shows slowing most prominent in the temporal regions and irregular background, but these changes are nonspecific, and EEG is generally not necessary.

7. The pathology consists of neuronal loss, deposition of amyloid plaques and neurofibrillary tangles, and secondary inflammatory changes. Research into deposition of these substances and the genetics of AD may offer effective treatment in the future. Patients may be eligible to participate in clinical trials directed at reducing amyloid deposition or neuronal loss.

8. There is a link between AD and apolipoprotein E (ApoE). There are three alleles for this gene, and the epsilon 4 allele is overrepresented in AD. However, the absence of an ApoE4 allele does not exclude the possibility that AD will be present pathologically; its absence also does not ensure that this is the correct diagnosis. Conversely, some subjects with an ApoE4 allele do not show symptoms of AD even after the age of 80 years.

9. For *treatment* cholinesterase inhibitors may provide tempo-rary improvement or stabilization of the disease. Tacrine has potential side effects of hepatic dysfunction and nausea and is used rarely. Donepezil is a cholinesterase inhibitor that is well tolerated and is used for symptomatic treatment of AD. Other cholinesterase inhibitors with modest efficacy include rivastigmine, metrifonate, and galantamine. Gas-trointestinal side effects are the most common adverse events with this class of medication. Selegiline and alpha-tocopherol may slow the progression of AD. Ginkgo biloba, a plant extract, has a modest effect on cognitive function in AD. Many other medications are being investigated for their ability to alter the course and ameliorate the symp-toms of this disorder.

10. Drugs to modify disruptive behavior include neuroleptics, anxiolytics, and antidepressants. These drugs should be used cautiously because patients in this age group often have adverse responses to these medications. For antidepressants, selective serotonin reuptake inhibitor medications are pre-ferred because of their low incidence of adverse side effects in the elderly. Trazodone may be used if there is disordered nighttime sleep. Buspirone may be effective for anxiety in patients with AD.

Note: A distinction needs to be made between minimal cog-nitive impairment (MCI) and dementia. MCI is a condition in which patients forget more readily than in the past but in which virtually all other cognitive functions are intact. About 10% to 20% of such patients go on to having a dementing disorder (usu-ally AD), but many may not progress at all.

Multi-Infarct Dementia

MID refers to dementia associated with multiple infarctions. It is sometimes difficult to separate clinically from AD and may be part of a "mixed" dementia (i.e., both AD and MID are present). Suggestive features include vascular risk factors, history of strokes, a stepwise progression, focal neurologic signs, pseudob-ulbar palsy, and MRI or CT changes of significant multifocal ischemic disease. MID may occur in patients treated inade-quately for hypertension and is therefore potentially pre-ventable. Furthermore, treatment of hypertension may prevent progression. Cholinesterase inhibitors may be helpful in the cognitive impairment of some patients with MID.

Creutzfeldt-Jakob Disease

Creutzfeldt-Jakob disease (CJD) is a rare, rapidly progressive disorder caused by a proteinaceous infectious agent (prion). The prion appears to be an abnormal conformation of a naturally occurring protein. A profound dementia, ataxia, myoclonic jerks, and sometimes visual loss and motor neuron changes occur. EEG may show periodic sharp and slow waves that assist in the diagnosis. Pathologically the brain shows spongiform changes with vacuoles. MRI may show characteristic T_2 image changes in the striatum in CJD. A spinal fluid assay for the 14-3-3 brain protein supports the diagnosis if positive, but it is not specific for CJD and is positive in other neurodegenerative disorders. Death occurs in many weeks to several months, and there is no effective treatment. Clinical trials of antiprotein aggregating compounds are under way based on positive results in animal models.

Pick's Disease

Pick's disease (frontotemporal dementia) resembles AD clinically but is quite rare and pathologically distinct. Personality changes, altered judgment, apathy, and prominent frontal release signs are more marked than in AD. Pathologically, Pick's disease affects frontal and temporal lobes more than parietal lobes. Many cases of primary progressive aphasia have Pick's type pathology at autopsy. Pick's is considered one of the frontotemporal dementias.

Huntington's Disease

Huntington's disease presents as an insidious intellectual decline associated with psychiatric symptoms and chorea. Dementia, personality, and emotional disorder may precede the chorea. Inheritance is autosomal dominant and involves a genetic abnormality on the short arm of chromosome 4. An excess of a trinucleotide repeat (CAG) at the huntingtin gene locus confers the disease, and an increased number of repeats is associated with earlier onset of the disease. Family history is usually positive but must be diligently explored. Genetic testing and counseling are available. Genetic testing should not be obtained without psychologic support to the patient and family by knowledgeable care providers.

Lewy Body Dementia

Lewy body dementia is a relatively recently recognized disorder that appears to be a common cause of dementia. In addition to the dementia, characteristic clinical features include fluctuations in the patient's cognitive or functional abilities, visual hallucinations, and prominent extrapyramidal signs. Extreme sensitivity to neuroleptic medications is characteristic. There are no specific diagnostic tests. Pathologically the disease is characterized by Lewy bodies (eosinophilic cytoplasmic inclusions in neurons) in the cortex and subcortex. The patient may have some response to cholinesterase inhibitors but tends to be less responsive to dopaminergic agents than are patients with Parkinson's disease.

LABORATORY WORKUP

A basic screen for dementia should include a complete blood count; urinalysis; measurement of electrolyte, calcium, blood urea nitrogen, vitamin B_{12}, and folate levels as well as sedimentation rate; liver function tests; thyroid function tests; serologic tests for syphilis (in endemic areas); HIV liter (where appropriate); drug levels (where appropriate); electrocardiogram, chest radiograph; CT scan or MRI of the brain; LP if chronic meningitis or opportunistic infection is suspected; and neuropsychologic testing (where appropriate).

With a careful history, physical examination, and the preceding studies, the etiology of dementia should become clear in most cases. If the diagnosis remains uncertain, other studies, such as arteriography or brain biopsy, are sometimes necessary. The extent of the workup depends on the patient's age and previous level of function. Remember, the primary goal of the workup of a patient with dementia is to find a treatable cause or a treatable component.

Guide the Patient and Family to Helpful Information and Resources

1. Provide referral to local support and information agencies.
2. Suggest several well-written books for the lay public with useful information about AD and other dementias and their treatment.

3. Consider daycare and respite-care programs.
4. Withdraw driving privileges if patients become disoriented in the house, get lost while walking outside or driving, or generally advance in their dementia

Suggested Reading

American College of Medical Genetics. Statement on use of Apolipoprotein E testing for Alzheimer disease. *JAMA* 1995;274:1627–1629.

Brown P. Infectious cerebral amyloidoses: Creutzfeldt-Jakob disease and the Gerstmann-Straussler-Scheinker syndrome. In: Morris JC, ed. *Handbook of dementing illnesses*. New York: Marcel Dekker, 1994: 353–376

Coker SB. The diagnosis of childhood degenerative disorders presenting as dementia in adults. *Neurology* 1991;41:794–798.

Folstein MF, Folstein SE, McHugh PR. "Mini-mental state": A practical method for grading the cognitive state of patients for the clinician. *J Psychiat Res* 1975;12:189–198.

Friedland RP. Alzheimer's disease: clinical features and differential diagnosis. *Neurology* 1993;43(suppl 4):S45–S51.

Geldmacher DS, Whitehouse PJ. Evaluation of dementia. *N Engl J Med* 1996;335:330–336.

Geldmacher DS, Whitehouse PJ. Differential diagnosis of Alzheimer's disease. *Neurology* 1997;48 (suppl 6):S2–S9.

Haywood FH. Transmissible spongiform encephalopathies. *N Engl J Med* 1997;337:1821–1828.

Hsich G, Kenney K, Gibbs CJ, et al. The 14-3-3 brain protein in cerebrospinal fluid as a marker for transmissible spongiform encephalopathies. *N Engl J Med* 1996;335:924–930.

Knapp MJ, Knopman DS, Solomon PR, et al. A 30-week randomized controlled trial of high-dose Tacrine in patients with Alzheimer's disease. *JAMA* 1994;271:985–991.

LeBars PL, Katz MM, Herman N, et al. A placebo-controlled, double-blind, randomized trial of an extract of Ginkgo Biloba for dementia. *JAMA* 1997;278:1327–1332.

McKeith IG, Galasko D, Kosaka K, et al. Consensus guidelines for the clinical and pathologic diagnosis of dementia with Lewy bodies (DLB): report of the consortium on DLB international workshop. *Neurology* 1996;47:1113–1124.

Mendez MF, Selwood A, Mastri AR, et al. Pick's disease versus Alzheimer's disease: a comparison of clinical characteristics. *Neurology* 1993:43: 289–292.

Neary D, Snowden JS, Gustafson L, et al. Frontotemporal lobar degeneration: a consensus on clinical diagnostic criteria. *Neurology* 1998;51: 1546–1554.

Rogers SL, Farlow MR, Doody RS, et al. A 24-week double-blind placebo controlled trial of donepezil in patients with Alzheimer's disease. Donepezil Study Group. *Neurology* 1998;50:136–145.

Sano M, Ernesto C, Thomas RG, et al. A controlled trial of selegiline, alpha-tocopherol, or both as treatment for Alzheimer's disease. *N Engl J Med* 1997;336:1216–1222.

Selkoe DJ. Alzheimer's disease: genes, proteins, and therapy. *Physiol Rev* 2001;81(2):741–766.

Chapter 20

Seizures and Epilepsy

Case

A 17-year-old senior in high school with no history of prenatal injury, febrile convulsions, head injury, or meningitis is being treated with valproic acid for seizures and has been seizure free for 1 year. At age 13, he had the first of three generalized tonic-clonic seizures. At age 15, he noticed that his body would jerk for a few minutes after awakening, and on one occasion this was followed by a convulsion. At age 16, he was noticed to stare from time to time in school. His electroencephalogram (EEG) shows generalized spike-and-wave activity.

Diagnosis

Juvenile myoclonic epilepsy with associated absence seizures.

A seizure reflects a transient neurologic symptom caused by the sudden abnormal discharge of a group of cerebral neurons. In general, seizures are a symptom of underlying brain disease—not a diagnosis. Epilepsy is the condition of repeated spontaneous and unprovoked seizures. Epilepsy has a variety of causes, both genetically determined and acquired.

TYPES OF SEIZURES

Seizures are categorized into two major types, depending on the presumed source: partial (focal) seizures or generalized seizures (Table 20.1). In partial (focal) seizures, the initial discharge

TABLE 20.1. International Classification of Epileptic Seizures

Partial Seizures (Begin Focally)	Generalized Seizures (Nonfocal)
Simple partial seizures	Absence
Complex partial seizures	Tonic
Partial seizures evolving into secondary generalized seizures	Clonic
	Atonic
	Myoclonic
	Tonic-clonic

(From Proposal for classification of epilepsies and epileptic syndromes. Commission on Classification and Terminology of the International League Against Epilepsy. *Epilepsia* 1985;26:268–278, with permission.)

comes from a specific part of the brain: temporal lobe, frontal lobe, motor strip, and so on. Such patients have symptoms depending on the involved area of cortex. Thus, patients whose seizures begin with their right hand shaking or with an aura of smelling "burned candy" have a partial seizure disorder, attributable to a lesion in the frontal or temporal lobe, respectively. Partial seizures with impairment of consciousness are known as complex partial seizures, to be distinguished from simple partial seizures, which have no such impairment of consciousness. Remember, a seizure can begin focally and then generalize. This may happen so quickly that it is impossible to see the focality clinically, and the patient can recall no aura. Nonetheless, the EEG usually shows the focality, and historical clues [brain tumor, arteriovenous malformation (AVM)] may suggest a focal origin. Partial seizure disorders are usually secondary to local pathology (e.g., trauma, tumor, vascular lesions, or congenital abnormalities).

It is important to recognize that partial complex seizures may be manifest only by unusual and paroxysmal changes in behavior, without loss of consciousness or convulsive motor activity. This is especially true in the elderly, in which the incidence of epilepsy is increasing dramatically and in which the manifestations of seizures can be unusual.

In *generalized seizures,* there are no focal sites of seizure origin. There is no aura, and there are no focal features during the seizure. Examples of generalized seizures include absence seizures (previously called petit mal) and idiopathic tonic-clonic seizures (previously called grand mal). A tonic-clonic seizure is a major motor seizure involving all extremities and having tonic (stiffening) and clonic (rhythmic jerking) movements. Myoclonic jerks (rapid individual muscle movements) also may be seen in primary generalized epilepsy, often as a syndrome in teenage years combined with absence seizures and rare tonic-clonic seizures (juvenile myoclonic epilepsy of Janz).

Note: Generalized tonic-clonic seizures may occur in normal individuals secondary to drug withdrawal, excessive sleep deprivation, brief episodes of hypotension (e.g., postsyncopal seizures), or metabolic factors (e.g., uremia, hypoglycemia). These are almost always generalized at onset but may be focal if the individual has an underlying focal neurologic lesion that is unrelated to the seizure. Individuals with these kinds of symptomatic seizures do not have epilepsy and usually are not treated for the seizures, but they may require treatment for the provocative medical condition responsible for the seizures. Seizures may follow unusual stress ("precipitated convulsions") and likewise are not considered epilepsy.

ESTABLISH WHETHER THE SEIZURE DISORDER IS FOCAL OR GENERALIZED

History

Is there a history of unusual behavior, with or without loss of consciousness, that is not explained by other medical diagnoses? Does the patient remember the event? Is there any retrograde amnesia? Is there confusion after the event?

1. Exactly how did the seizure start? Find a witness. Did the head and eyes turn? Were there other focal features? Was there an aura?
2. At what age did the seizures begin? This is important. Primary generalized seizures rarely begin before age 3 years or after age 18. "Absence seizures" that begin during adulthood are usually complex partial seizures of temporal lobe origin.
3. Is there a family history of seizures? This may be present in both types but is more characteristic of generalized seizure disorders.
4. Was there focal trauma at birth or during an accident (head trauma)? Is there a history of a previous neurologic insult (e.g., stroke, encephalitis, meningitis)?

5. Does the patient have abdominal pains, nausea, dizziness, behavioral disturbances, or automatisms (frequent features of temporal lobe epilepsy)? Are there déjà vu phenomena (vivid memories of prior experiences)? Does the patient smell an odd smell for a few moments (a common symptom of seizures from the mesial temporal lobe)?

6. Have there been brief staring spells not followed by postictal confusion or fatigue (absence seizures)?

7. Is there a history of recent drug or alcohol ingestion or withdrawal or of excessive sleep deprivation?

8. Is there an underlying risk factor for seizure present (e.g., human immunodeficiency virus infection or diabetes)? Has there been travel to the Southwest or South America (cysticercosis)?

9. Is there a history of cardiac arrhythmias or hypotension that could account for a loss of consciousness?

Examination

1. Look for postictal paralysis (Todd's paralysis) by checking for asymmetry of reflexes, hemiparesis, an up-going toe, or hemiparetic posturing of a foot (averted).

2. Are the eyes tonically deviated during the seizure? For example, a left hemisphere seizure usually drives the eyes to the right.

3. Look for asymmetry of fingernail, toe, and limb size (a clue to early damage to the contralateral hemisphere).

4. Absence seizures (a primary generalized seizure of childhood) can be precipitated by hyperventilation. Have the patient breathe deeply for 5 minutes, and watch for a brief, transient cessation of activity and "glassy stare."

5. Examine the skin carefully. Neurocutaneous disorders, such as neurofibromatosis, tuberous sclerosis, and Sturge-Weber disease, may present with seizures.

LABORATORY AIDS IN DIAGNOSIS

1. In addition to baseline laboratory studies (including glucose, blood urea nitrogen, calcium, sodium), perform an EEG and a magnetic resonance imaging (MRI) scan or computed tomography (CT) scan (MRI is more sensitive than a CT scan in locating the etiology in focal seizures) for any unex-

plained first seizure. Perform a lumbar puncture (LP) if there is any suspicion of infection. If the seizure was focal or if a mass lesion is suspected, be sure there is no papilledema or midline shift before doing the LP.

2. Obtain a sleep-deprived EEG if a focal seizure disorder is suspected. Frequently, it will bring out the spike focus. In some cases, the spike focus can be seen only with special (e.g., anterior temporal, nasopharyngeal, or sphenoidal) EEG leads.

3. MRI is accurate in detecting small tumors, focal gliosis, cortical dysgenesis, and mesial temporal sclerosis, all of which may cause partial seizures. Coronal thin slices through the temporal lobes using fluid-attenuation inversion recovery (FLAIR) sequences increase the yield of MRI in focal epilepsies.

Note: It may be difficult to differentiate between absence and complex partial seizures. Remember that absence seizures have no warning (aura), are abrupt in onset, and are brief (last seconds); the patient has a prompt return to consciousness. Also, absence seizures are characterized by a 3 Hz spike-and-wave EEG pattern and almost always begin in childhood.

WHAT ETIOLOGIC FACTORS ARE INVOLVED?

Metabolic factors, such as hypoglycemia, hypocalcemia, or electrolyte imbalance, may play a role at any age. Other "metabolic" causes include uremia, hepatic failure, and hypoxia. Hypothyroidism can worsen a preexisting seizure disorder.

Drug withdrawal (from alcohol, barbiturates, and other sedatives) is a common cause of seizures in adults. Alcohol withdrawal seizures occur 12 to 48 hours after the cessation of drinking (see Chapter 27). Alcoholics with posttraumatic epilepsy secondary to frequent falls may have an exacerbation of seizures when intoxicated.

Exacerbation of a known seizure disorder is common. Persons with a controlled seizure disorder who come to the hospital because of a recurrence usually (a) have not been taking their medication (draw blood level); (b) have been drinking; or (c) have an intercurrent infection. Change in lifestyle, emotional stress, menses, or sleep deprivation also may exacerbate seizures. Temporarily increase the medication if seizures occur during a period of intercurrent infection. Reevaluate anyone with a well-controlled seizure disorder that worsens with no apparent cause. More than half of the cases of *posttraumatic epilepsy* develop during the first year after injury, and more than 80% develop by 4 years. There occasionally are delayed cases. Penetrating injuries of the dura, cerebral hemorrhage and contusion, brain infection, focal neurologic signs, and prolonged coma all increase the risk of epilepsy. A seizure immediately after head injury is not a specific risk factor for epilepsy, but seizures within the first week increase that risk. *Subdural hematoma* can be associated with seizures and must be considered in an alcoholic with new onset of seizures.

Etiology as related to *age of onset* is as follows:

- Infancy and childhood: birth injury, congenital malformations, infections, trauma, metabolic disorders, genetic, idiopathic
- Adolescence: idiopathic, genetic, trauma, drug-related
- Young adult: trauma, alcohol, neoplasm, drug-related, AVM
- Middle age: neoplasm, alcohol, vascular disease, trauma, AVM
- Late life (older than age 65 years): vascular disease, neoplasm, associated with dementia

Note: Idiopathic or primary generalized epilepsy usually is apparent by age 18. Seizures beginning after age 18 usually are caused by a focal process, metabolic derangement, or withdrawal state. Neoplasm is of prime concern during all of adult life. After age 65 years, vascular disease (stroke) is the most common cause of a first seizure.

Genetic etiologies for seizures are important in infants and young adults. Epilepsies previously labeled idiopathic now are known to be genetic. Genetic transmission of seizures can be autosomal dominant, autosomal recessive, or mitochondrial. Examples of genetic epilepsies include childhood absence epilepsy and juvenile myoclonic epilepsy.

Sudden Unexpected Death in Epilepsy

Sudden unexpected death in epilepsy (SUDEP) occurs in approximately 1 per 300 patients with epilepsy per year in adulthood. These deaths do not occur in the context of trauma, drowning, or status epilepticus. SUDEP is common with severe epilepsy and in patients who have poorly controlled epilepsy. SUDEP occurs more commonly in males than females and usually in the young adult years. SUDEP may occur with changes in seizure medications or with poor compliance with antiepileptic drugs (AEDs).

TREATMENT TIPS

Drugs for Partial Seizure Disorders

Treatment is initiated with a single agent. Patients who fail the first agent are less likely to be completely controlled with subsequent medications. Carbamazepine, oxcarbazepine, phenytoin, or valproic acid is the drug of first choice used to treat adults with partial seizures. As a rule, do not use two drugs unless one drug in adequate dosage (check blood levels) does not control the seizures. Newer drugs such as gabapentin, levetiracetam, lamotrigine, tiagabine, topiramate, and zonisamide are available as add-on medications for the treatment of complex partial seizures but have a higher cost than other AEDs. Many of these medications are used as monotherapy despite being primarily tested as add-on therapy in clinical trials. Many of the newer AEDs are better tolerated and have different side effect profiles than the older drugs. For example, many do not induce liver enzymes and therefore will not interfere with oral contraceptive medication or warfarin. It is best to tailor the choice of first drug to the patient.

Drugs for Primary Generalized Seizure Disorders

Valproic acid, carbamazepine, and phenytoin are first-line medications for primary generalized seizures. Alternatives include lamotrigine, levetiracetam, and topiramate. Ethosuximide may be used alone for absence seizures but only if there are no associated tonic-clonic seizures (it has no activity against these). Valproic acid is useful in absence seizures, especially when there *are* associated tonic-clonic seizures.

Convulsive Status Epilepticus

Convulsive status epilepticus has been defined as continuous seizure activity for 30 minutes or recurrent seizures for 30 minutes without resumption of consciousness. Evidence suggests that even shorter periods of continuous seizures can be deleterious to the brain, and the definition of "status epilepticus" is undergoing some revision. Convulsive status epilepticus, whatever its definition, remains a true medical emergency.

1. Maintain airway, administer O_2, prevent aspiration, and maintain blood pressure (ABCs). While doing so, obtain a brief history from family or friends and perform a brief examination (e.g., is the patient a known epileptic who stopped taking medication or developed an infection?).

2. Draw blood to check glucose, electrolytes, calcium, magnesium, complete blood count, and toxic screens. Check AED levels if appropriate. Check oxygenation. Start an intravenous (IV) line, and administer 100 mg thiamine followed by 50 mL of 50% glucose.

3. Administer either 0.1 mg/kg lorazepam at 2 mg/minute or 0.2 mg/kg of diazepam at 5 mg/minute intravenously. Either drug may cause respiratory arrest, especially in patients who previously have been administered barbiturates, and thus should be used cautiously. These drugs stop seizures but have a relatively short duration of action and need to be followed by a second AED for longer-term control.

4. Phenytoin or fos-phenytoin may be used for status epilepticus (phenytoin or phenytoin equivalents 15 to 18 mg/kg intravenously over 30 to 45 minutes). Either may be increased to 30 mg/kg if seizures continue. Hypotension can occur if phenytoin is given too quickly. Thus, do not administer phenytoin faster than 50 mg/minute and have blood pressure and electrocardiogram monitored periodically during IV administration. Fos-phenytoin may be administered up to 150 mg/minute but is metabolized to phenytoin so that the onset of action is equivalent to that of phenytoin. Use phenytoin cautiously in patients with heart disease. In those with conduction defects, phenytoin is relatively contraindicated. For administration, phenytoin is given intravenously in normal saline; it will precipitate in dextrose solutions. Fos-phenytoin is a dilantin prodrug. It may be given intramuscularly. It appears to have less cardiotoxicity. It must be converted into phenytoin to be active; thus, its mode of action is similar to that of phenytoin.

5. If benzodiazepines and phenytoin/fos-phenytoin are ineffective in status epilepticus, other agents may be added. If phenobarbital is given after phenytoin, it should be administered cautiously at a dose of 100 mg/minute intravenously, up to 20 mg/kg. Respiration and blood pressure must be watched carefully, particularly if the patient has received benzodiazepines, and intubation usually is required.

6. Refractory status epilepticus may be difficult to control and has a high mortality. Medications that have been tried in small series include pentobarbital, high-dose phenobarbital, midazolam infusions, propofol infusions, and other medications. Treatment of refractory status requires intubation for respiratory insufficiency and airway control, careful intensive care unit monitoring, preferably continuous EEG monitoring, and neurologic consultation. Vasopressors may be necessary.

7. When it proves difficult to control status epilepticus, there is often an underlying metabolic disorder (e.g., hyponatremia, hypoglycemia) or structural lesion (e.g., subdural, meningitis). Imaging and LP should be considered in this setting.

8. The most likely etiology of status epilepticus if there is no history of seizures is stroke, tumor, or trauma. If there is a history of seizures, an intercurrent illness or noncompliance with medication is usually responsible.

Note: Mortality from status epilepticus increases dramatically with duration of status. Early effective treatment is critical.

THERAPEUTIC AGENTS

Phenytoin (Dilantin)

1. The average adult dose is 300 to 400 mg/day.

2. Therapeutic blood levels are 10 to 20 μg/mL; levels should be monitored in any patient who has not achieved good seizure control by taking phenytoin or other anticonvulsant medications. Some patients require a level outside the standard therapeutic range for optimal control. It may be useful to obtain a level when the patient is doing well to assess an optimal dose for that patient.

3. Administered orally, it may take 3 or 5 days to achieve a steady state; IV administration in adequate doses gives thera-

peutic levels within an hour. Patients also may be given loading doses orally (e.g., 500 mg initially, followed by 300 mg 2 hours later, and 200 to 400 mg 2 hours later followed by daily maintenance doses). Intramuscular phenytoin is not absorbed evenly, causes muscle necrosis, and should be avoided. Fos-phenytoin may be given intravenously or intramuscularly.

4. Nystagmus on lateral gaze is a good clinical sign that the patient is taking the medication. Ataxia of gait and lethargy are common manifestations of toxicity. Irritability and diplopia are other dose-related symptoms.

5. Phenytoin is metabolized by the liver, so one usually can give regular doses to patients who have renal disease or are in renal failure. It is of value to check the level of free (unbound, active) phenytoin in these patients and in pregnant patients taking phenytoin.

6. A morbilliform rash occurs in approximately 4% of patients. If this occurs, it is best to stop the phenytoin use and choose an alternate anticonvulsant.

7. Other side effects include hirsutism, gingival hypertrophy, megaloblastic anemia, osteomalacia, lymphadenopathy, and lupuslike syndrome. A teratogenic effect of phenytoin has been reported. With long-term use, a mild distal polyneuropathy may occur.

8. Warfarin and isoniazid enhance the action of phenytoin, and INR may be altered by phenytoin in patients on warfarin. Chronic administration of barbiturates may decrease blood phenytoin levels. Patients taking phenytoin may have factitiously low thyroid function test levels.

9. Phenytoin levels may increase suddenly when its receptor sites are saturated. Thus, when a patient whose seizures are not yet controlled has a blood level in the therapeutic range, use 30 mg capsules to titrate the dose or alternate 300 and 400 mg daily.

10. Despite its longstanding role in epilepsy, phenytoin is being used less and less, primarily because of its side effect profile and its complex pharmacology.

Carbamazepine

1. The carbamazepine dosage in adults is 600 to 1,200 mg/day in three divided doses. Long-acting forms (Tegretol-XR or

Carbatrol) allow for twice-a-day dosing. A gradual dose escalation avoids many of the problems of initiating carbamazepine, including gastrointestinal upset, and those related to the delayed induction of hepatic enzymes.

2. Therapeutic blood levels are 4 to 12 μg/mL.

3. Toxic side effects include leukopenia, thrombocytopenia, hepatic dysfunction, hyponatremia, and rashes. Hyponatremia may be renally mediated. Dose-related side effects include sedation, ataxia, diplopia, and blurred vision.

4. Carbamazepine is effective for focally originating seizures (drug of choice) and tonic-clonic seizures.

5. Occasionally, carbamazepine may exacerbate absence seizures in patients being treated for primary generalized tonic-clonic seizures.

6. Neural tube defects are reported in 1% of children born to mothers who are taking carbamazepine.

7. Watch for a dramatic increase in carbamazepine levels with concurrent use of erythromycin or propoxyphene, which blocks hepatic metabolism of this medication.

Valproic Acid

1. The initial dose is 15 mg/kg. Titration up to 60 mg/kg is necessary in some cases.

2. Therapeutic blood levels are 50 to 100 μg/mL, although blood levels may correlate poorly with clinical response.

3. Valproic acid is most effective in absence, myoclonic, and akinetic seizures and primary generalized epilepsies.

4. Toxic effects include gastrointestinal disturbances and sedation (especially if the dose is built up rapidly), ataxia, liver dysfunction, thrombocytopenia, and pancreatitis. Hair loss, weight gain, and tremor are noticeable side effects in some patients. Hepatic failure may be seen in children younger than age 2 years who are treated with polypharmacy; it is rare in adults.

5. Teratogenic effects with neural tube defects occur in 1% to 2% of children born to mothers taking valproic acid. Thus, this drug should be avoided in pregnant women, if possible.

6. Interactions with other anticonvulsant medications include increased phenobarbital levels and increased free phenytoin levels.

Oxcarbazepine

1. Oxcarbazepine is closely related to carbamazepine and has been used in Europe since the early 1990s.
2. It may be used as monotherapy for partial and secondarily generalized seizures.
3. It may aggravate absence or myoclonic seizures.
4. The usual total adult dose is 1,200 to 2,400 mg/day, with the drug given twice a day.
5. Adverse effects are similar to carbamazepine. Leukopenia occurs less frequently than with carbamazepine.
6. It is generally well tolerated with a favorable side effect profile.

Gabapentin

1. For dosage, begin with 300 mg the first day, increasing to 900 mg/day in three divided doses. Some patients are treated with up to 5,400 mg/day for refractory seizures.
2. Gabapentin is used primarily as an add-on medication for partial seizures, although it has been shown to be effective in monotherapy.
3. Dose-related side effects include dizziness, somnolence, and fatigue.
4. Gabapentin is not metabolized significantly, remains unbound, and has virtually no interactions with other medications. It is excreted by the kidney and has an excellent safety profile.
5. Gabapentin has moderate efficacy in the treatment of partial seizures.

Lamotrigine

1. Very gradually titrate (over weeks) to a dose of 200 to 600 mg/day in two divided doses. A lower dose and slower titration is used in patients taking valproic acid.
2. Lamotrigine is an effective medication for partial and generalized seizures and may be used as an add-on drug for partial epilepsies. It has a broad spectrum of efficacy for epilepsy.
3. Side effects include skin rash, somnolence, and dizziness. Hypersensitivity rash is most common, with rapid titration and rare cases of Stevens-Johnson syndrome being reported.

4. The half-life is 12 hours with enzyme-inducing medications, 24 hours with monotherapy, and 48 to 72 hours with concomitant valproic acid.

Felbamate

1. Aplastic anemia and hepatic failure have made felbamate a medication to be used only by neurologists experienced with its toxicity, usually after failure of other seizure medication.
2. It is approved for treatment of partial epilepsy and for patients with Lennox-Gastaut syndrome.
3. It is used alone or in combination with other AEDs.

Tiagabine

1. Tiagabine is used as an add-on medication for partial seizures.
2. Tiagabine is generally well tolerated. High doses often cause sedation and dizziness.
3. Its efficacy is relatively modest.

Topiramate

1. Topiramate is an add-on medication for partial seizures and secondary generalized seizures. Significant side effects include somnolence, blurred vision, and ataxia.
2. Effective doses are between 200 to 400 mg/day using bid dosing.
3. Side effects include fatigue, gastrointestinal upset, dizziness, impaired thinking, and irritability.
4. Renal calculi occur in 1% to 3% of patients; thus, adequate fluid intake should be encouraged.

Levetiracetam

1. Levetiracetam is approved as an add-on medication for partial seizures.
2. Usual dosages are 1,000 to 3,000 mg/day in bid dosing.
3. Side effects include somnolence, irritability, asthenia, and dizziness.
4. Drug interactions are limited.
5. Safety appears to be excellent with this medication, and efficacy is good.

Zonisamide

1. Zonisamide is approved as an add-on medication for partial seizures and secondary generalized seizures. It also may be effective in generalized seizures.
2. Adverse reactions include drowsiness, ataxia, loss of appetite, and slowing of cognition.
3. Renal stones occur in 1% to 2% of patients.
4. The risk of renal stones is greater with a family history.
5. Zonisamide is contraindicated in patients with sulfonamide hypersensitivity.

Note: Phenobarbital has been used in the control of epilepsy for many years. However, it is no longer a primary option because of its sedative effect, cognitive impairment in children, and the risk of withdrawal seizures.

OTHER ISSUES IN THE MANAGEMENT OF SEIZURES

Education

Treatment includes education of the patient. Emphasize that epilepsy is not a mental illness; it is the condition of having seizures. Discuss driving (guidelines are determined state by state) and avoidance of precipitating factors (e.g., drugs and alcohol, sleep deprivation). Emphasize compliance with medication regimens. Discuss issues of employment and safety, and teach the family simple first-aid tips. Provide educational materials, and refer the patient to the local epilepsy society for information and support. Remember, epilepsy is a chronic condition and a well-educated patient is a therapeutic ally.

Treatment of the First Seizure

Not all patients with a first seizure require treatment. Overall about 50% of patients with a first seizure will have a recurrence in the next 3 to 5 years. Factors that increase the risk of recurrence include structural brain lesions, an EEG with a definite epileptiform pattern, a history of a prior brain insult, and status epilepticus as a first seizure. Such patients usually are treated. Patients with a seizure in the setting of drug or alcohol withdrawal, with an acute illness, immediately after a concussion, or with excessive sleep deprivation usually do not need treatment. Patients with two or three unprecipitated seizures have a high risk of recurrence and should be treated. Patients without structural lesions, with a normal EEG, and with a normal neurologic examination usually do not need treatment after a first seizure.

Discontinuing Antiepileptic Drugs in Seizure-Free Patients

Guidelines by the American Academy of Neurology suggest that patients who are seizure free for 2 to 5 years, with a single type of partial or generalized seizure, normal neurologic examination and IQ, and a normalized EEG, have the greatest chance for successful drug withdrawal. Such patients have a 60% to 70% chance of successful withdrawal. The risks of drug withdrawal should be discussed with the patient, and driving should be restricted during the first few months after tapering off the medication.

Seizures and Pregnancy

The care of the pregnant patient with epilepsy should be undertaken by physicians experienced in this area. Prenatal folate vitamins will decrease the risk of teratogenesis (the dose is at least 1 mg/day). This may be necessary within the first month of pregnancy, usually before a woman is aware she is pregnant. Thus, many neurologists prescribe folate for all women with epilepsy in the childbearing years. In general, patients taking AEDs have a slightly increased risk of complications of pregnancy and minor and major teratogenic defects of the fetus. Carbamazepine and valproic acid cause an increased risk of neural tube defects, but it is unclear whether higher doses of folate (e.g., 5 mg/day) will reduce this risk. In general, the best AED to be used in a pregnant patient with epilepsy is that drug most likely to best control the seizures. Many AEDs have altered pharmacokinetics in pregnancy and need careful monitoring. Withdrawing medication before pregnancy should be done only in patients considered likely to remain seizure free; withdrawing medication after conception and pregnancy are established adds the risk of seizure to the risk of teratogenesis. Trying to reduce to a single medication before conception is reasonable. Certain AEDs make the risk of neonatal hemorrhage greater and may be prevented by vitamin K administered to the mother during the last month of pregnancy and to the newborn. Approximately 90% to 95% of children born to mothers with epilepsy are normal.

Seizure Surgery

Surgery is being used more commonly for the treatment of medically intractable epilepsy by the excision of epileptogenic cortex. This therapeutic option usually is considered after 1 to 2 years of medication trials do not control seizures and in cases in which a seizure focus is accessible for surgical treatment. The results are variable, depending on individual circumstances. For patients with intractable temporal lobe epilepsy who have an early risk factor (e.g., meningitis, prolonged febrile seizures, head trauma) and an MRI that demonstrates unilateral hippocampal sclerosis, as many as 75% to 85% will become seizure free, and many of the rest will have a major reduction of seizures. For individuals who do not fit the "ideal" conditions, seizure-free rates after temporal lobectomy approach 50%. For individuals with neocortical lesions, results are variable, depending on the nature of the underlying lesion and its location. The implantation of a vagal nerve stimulator has been associated with cessation of seizures in approximately 10% of patients with intractable epilepsy and may reduce seizure frequency in another 30% to 40% of patients.

Suggested Reading

Bergin AM, Connolly M. New antiepileptic drug therapies. *Neurol Clin* 2002;20(4):1163–1182.

Blume WT. Diagnosis and management of epilepsy. *CMAJ* 2003;168(4): 441–448.

Brodie MJ, French J. Management of epilepsy in adolescents and adults. *Lancet* 2000;356:323–329.

Dichter M, Buchhalter J. The genetic epilepsies. In: Rosenberg R, Prusiner S, DiMauro S, eds. *The molecular and genetic basis of neurological and psychiatric diseases*. Boston: Butterworth, 2003.

Generalized idiopathic epilepsies. Available at *http://www.mynchen.demon.co.uk*. Accessed October 8, 2003.

Greenwood RS. Adverse effects of antiepileptic drugs. *Epilepsia* 2000; 41(suppl2):S42–S52.

Langan Y. Sudden unexpected death in epilepsy (SUDEP); risk factors and case control studies. *Seizure* 2000;9:179–183.

Liporace J, D'Abreu A. Epilepsy and women's health. *Mayo Clin Proc* 2003;78:497–506.

Manno EM. New management strategies in the treatment of status epilepticus. *Mayo Clin Proc* 2003;78(4):508–518.

Nguyen DK, Spencer SS. Recent advances in the treatment of epilepsy. *Arch Neurol* 2003;60:929–935.

Ruegg S, Dichter MA. Diagnosis and treatment of nonconvulsive status epilepticus in an intensive care unit setting. *Curr Treat Options Neurol* 2003;5:93–110.

Sheth RD, Stafstrom CE. Intractable pediatric epilepsy: vagal nerve stimulation and the ketogenic diet. *Neurol Clin* 2002;20(4):1183–1194.

Thomas RJ. Seizures and epilepsy in the elderly. *Arch Intern Med* 1997; 157:605–617.

Wiebe S, Blume WT, Girvin JP, et al. A randomized controlled trial of surgery for temporal-lobe epilepsy. *N Engl J Med* 2001;345:311–318.

Yerby MS. Clinical care of pregnant women with epilepsy: neural tube defects and folic acid supplementation. *Epilepsia* 2003;44(Suppl 3): 33–40.

Chapter 21

Multiple Sclerosis and Related Disorders

Case

A 34-year-old woman experiences a sudden loss of vision in the left eye that lasts for 2 months, with spontaneous resolution. Three years later, she notices numbness ascending to the waistline that partially resolves after 6 weeks. The following year she develops unsteady gait and slurred speech over a 1-week period. She is treated with intravenous (IV) methylprednisolone and improves. Her magnetic resonance imaging (MRI) scan shows periventricular lesions, and her cerebrospinal fluid (CSF) has increased immunoglobulin G (IgG) and oligoclonal bands.

Diagnosis

Relapsing remitting multiple sclerosis (MS).

Multiple Sclerosis (MS) is a relapsing-progressive disorder that affects the white matter of the central nervous system (CNS; brain and spinal cord). It is an inflammatory disease in which lymphocytes and macrophages damage the myelin sheath and also may cause axonal damage. It is more common in women and usually begins from ages 20 to 40 years, although it may begin after age 40. MS generally is considered a cell-mediated autoimmune disease directed against myelin components triggered in some fashion by a viral infection. Despite many attempts, an infectious agent has not been identified in MS, and MS is not considered an infectious disease.

CLASSIFICATION OF MS

Major Categories

1. *Relapsing-remitting.* Patients have discrete motor, sensory, cerebellar, or visual attacks that come on over a 1 to 2 week period and resolve over a 4 to 8 week period with or without corticosteroid treatment. Patients in this category often return to their preattack baseline.
2. *Transitional.* Patients have attacks but do not return to their baseline and accumulate stepwise disability. They may have a progressive component in their illness. This is a transitional stage between relapsing-remitting and progressive and may be classified as a more severe form of relapsing-remitting disease. These patients may be unresponsive to medication for relapsing-remitting MS and may benefit from more aggressive immunosuppression.
3. *Secondary progressive.* Gradual neurologic deterioration occurs in a patient who previously had relapsing-remitting MS.
4. *Primary progressive.* Patients follow a continuous slowly progressive course from the onset, usually with spinal cord involvement without exacerbations.

Rarer Categories

1. *Benign* MS: patients with mild exacerbations who never develop major exacerbations or disability symptoms
2. *Progressive relapsing*: gradual neurologic deterioration from the onset with subsequent superimposed exacerbations
3. *Fulminant*: rapid severe progression with relapses over a period of months

SIGNS AND SYMPTOMS

Signs and symptoms occur in multiple anatomic areas of brain and spinal cord affected by the disease.
    Common symptoms include the following:

■ Sensory (numbness, tingling, heaviness in an extremity, sensory level)
■ Visual (visual loss, color vision change, field defects)

- Brainstem (diplopia, dizziness, difficulty swallowing or speaking)
- Motor (weakness, spasticity, cramping)
- Cerebellar (ataxia of gait or of an extremity)
- Bowel and bladder dysfunction
- Cognitive complaints (even when neurologic symptoms are minimal)

  Common signs include the following:

- Corticospinal tract (weakness, spasticity, hyperreflexia, asymmetric reflexes, up-going toes)
- Sensory (vibration loss, decreased pin sense, sensory level)
- Brainstem (nystagmus, internuclear ophthalmoplegia, facial weakness)
- Optic nerve (loss of visual acuity, central scotomas, loss of color vision, optic nerve atrophy, afferent pupillary defect)
- Tremor

Note: Heat may worsen the symptoms by altering axonal conduction. Transient episodes of neurologic dysfunction (tonic spasms) may occur and last seconds or minutes.

DIAGNOSIS

The diagnosis of MS is based primarily on clinical findings reflecting involvement of multiple sites in the brain or spinal cord occurring at different times—"multiple lesions in time and space" and an abnormal MRI scan. MRI is the most important laboratory test and often shows multiple areas of white matter change in the periventricular white matter, corpus callosum, brainstem, and spinal cord. Active MS lesions enhance with gadolinium. CSF shows indication of an inflammatory process with mild pleocytosis and mild protein alteration, increased IgG/albumin ratio and IgG synthesis index, and oligoclonal banding. Evoked potentials (especially those that are visually evoked) are often abnormal and reflect areas of white matter demyelination. Clinically definite MS is defined as two attacks and clinical evidence of two separate lesions. In one study, 93% of such patients had abnormal MRIs, 87% had abnormal CSF, and 81% had abnormal visual evoked responses. MS also can be diagnosed in patients who have one attack or progressive disease from the onset and clinical or laboratory evidence of a second lesion in the CNS as defined by the McDonald MS diagnostic criteria.

MRI in MS. Based on MRI, it is now clear that subclinical MS activity occurs when patients appear to be in remission. The presence of disease activity is seen by newly appearing white matter lesions and lesions that enhance with gadolinium. Although imperfect, an active MRI and increasing T2 lesion level correlate with attacks and disability. Thus the MRI is becoming more important for treatment decisions (see later).

DIFFERENTIAL DIAGNOSIS

White matter lesions may be seen in a variety of disorders other than MS.

1. *Acute demyelinating encephalomyelitis.* A monophasic demyelinating illness may develop after immunizations or viral illnesses. This is usually of rapid onset with severe symptoms, fever, and confusion. Treatment is with high-dose steroids.
2. *Vasculitis.* Patients with vasculitis related to disorders such as meningovascular syphilis, Sjögren's syndrome, lupus erythematosus, Behçet's disease, Wegener's granulomatosis, and isolated CNS vasculitis may present with an MS-like picture. Asking about the features of the systemic disease and watching for atypical MRI or clinical appearance are helpful in diagnosis.
3. *Lyme disease.* Rarely, infections of the CNS may present like MS but usually have a different CSF and clinical picture. For example, in Lyme disease the typical skin rash, a meningitis presentation, or the presentation of radiculopathy would discriminate it from MS.
4. *Structural lesions.* Structural lesions such as cervical spondylosis, spinal cord tumor, or posterior fossa tumor may mimic MS. These abnormalities are identified by imaging the affected part of the nervous system.
5. B_{12} *deficiency.* B_{12} deficiency may cause white matter disease and spinal cord disease but usually as a monophasic illness or progressive illness.
6. *Dysmyelinating diseases and CADASIL* (Cerebral Autosomal Dominant Arteriopathy with Subcortical Infarcts and Leukoencephalopathy).

TREATMENT

Treatment of MS involves three components: (a) disease-modifying therapy directed at the immune system and (b) symptomatic therapy directed at improving nervous system function (e.g., spasticity).

Disease-Modifying Therapy

Several treatments have been shown to affect the course of the disease and are available to the physician. A hierarchy of therapies are given, depending on the stage and severity of the illness.

Most disease-modifying therapies decrease interferon gamma (IFN-γ) secretion. Some also induce the secretion of antiinflammatory cytokines such as interleukin-4 (IL-4), IL-10, and transforming growth factor beta (TGF-β). Drugs also may affect trafficking or migration of cells into the CNS.

1. *Acute attacks*, if mild, may not require treatment. If they affect function in a significant way, they may be treated with a short course of IV corticosteroids. Indications for treatment of a relapse include functionally disabling symptoms with objective evidence of neurologic impairment. The most commonly used regimen is a 3-day to 7-day course (1,000 mg/day) of IV methylprednisolone given without a prednisone taper.

2. *Relapsing-remitting disease.* Two forms of recombinant interferon beta (β-1a and 1b) and glatiramer acetate are approved for the treatment of *relapsing-remitting MS*. Interferon β-1b is given subcutaneously as every other day injections. Interferon β-1a is given as three weekly subcutaneous injections or as a weekly intramuscular injection, and glatiramer acetate is given as a daily subcutaneous injection. Side effects of interferon β include injection site reactions, influenzalike symptoms, and worsening of preexisting depression. The choice between the different interferon preparations depends on the patient and individual physician. The most common side effects of glatiramer acetate are mild injection site reactions and in some patients unexplained reactions involving episodes of flushing, chest tightness, shortness of breath, and palpitations. The choice of beginning a relapsing-remitting patient with interferon β versus glatiramer acetate has not been resolved.

Patients with depression, those early in their course, or those who cannot tolerate interferon β are often preferentially treated with glatiramer acetate. There is no consensus on which interferon to use. There is some evidence that higher doses of interferon may be more efficacious. It is recommended that all patients with relapsing-remitting MS be placed on some form of immunomodulatory therapy.

3. Patients with relapsing-remitting disease who are *nonresponders to βinterferon or glatiramer acetate* may be treated with the other medication ("rescue therapy"), depending on how active the disease has become. Nonresponders include those with continued attacks, increasing disability, and new disease activity on MRI. Drugs used as "rescue" therapy include IV pulse methylprednisolone and immunosuppressant drugs such as pulse cyclophosphamide and mitoxantrone. Clinical trials are under way testing several new immunomodulatory agents that can be used as "rescue therapy" or as primary therapy.

4. *Progressive MS.* Treatment directed at the *progressive phase of MS* is more difficult because the disease tends to become worse once the progressive stage has been initiated. B interferon has been shown to have an effect on patients with secondary progressive MS who continue to have attacks. Other drugs in use include cyclophosphamide, methotrexate, and mitoxantrone, depending on the type of progressive disease and how long the patient has been progressive. Cyclophosphamide may be given in an outpatient regimen similar to its use in lupus nephritis. It has become increasingly recognized that a degenerative component exists in MS, especially in later progressive stages, and immunomodulatory and immunosuppressive therapy may not be effective for this degenerative phase of the illness.

Please note:

1. *Optic neuritis.* This may occur during the course of MS or may be one of the initial symptoms. A recent trial of optic neuritis demonstrated that patients treated with oral prednisone alone were more likely to suffer recurrent episodes of optic neuritis as compared to those treated with methylprednisolone followed by oral prednisone. These results now make IV methylprednisolone the primary treatment used for

optic neuritis. Furthermore, as part of the optic neuritis study, it was found that treatment with a 3-day course of high-dose methylprednisolone reduced the rate of development of MS over a 2-year period. The protective effect was most apparent in patients at highest risk for MS—those with multiple focal brain MRI abnormalities. Patients treated with pulse IV methylprednisolone must be monitored for decreased bone density. Anaphylactoid reactions and arrhythmias also may occur.

2. *Fulminating disability.* An open study of plasmapheresis in acute episodes of fulminant CNS inflammatory demyelination showed marked improvement in patients who did not benefit from a course of high-dose IV methylprednisolone and appears to be an important therapeutic option for this rare subset of patients. The patient also may be treated with IV cyclophosphamide.

3. *Primary progressive MS.* This form of MS is difficult to treat and may represent a different pathologic process. Treatment with IV methylprednisolone or methotrexate often is attempted.

4. *Pregnancy.* Attacks of MS usually are decreased in frequency during pregnancy but are increased slightly in the postpartum period.

5. *Paroxysmal tonic seizures.* These seizures usually last 1 to 2 minutes and occur several times per day. The patient may confuse them with MS attacks. They consist of paresthesiae or pain in the face or a limb, followed by painful tonic contraction. Another paroxysmal symptom consists of dysarthria and ataxia, usually unilateral limb ataxia, although gait also may be affected. These episodes are also short lived (often less than 1 minute) and can occur several times per hour. Paroxysmal phenomena typically subside after a period of weeks. They likely are caused by ephaptic transmission of nerve impulses at sites of previous disease activity. Low doses of carbamazepine, phenytoin, or baclofen are usually effective and can be tapered after several weeks.

Symptomatic Therapy

1. *Spasticity.* Lioresal, Valium, and tizanidine are all effective antispasticity agents in MS. Regular exercise and stretching

are useful. For selected patients, an intrathecal pump of Lioresal is effective with a low side effect profile.

2. *Pain.* Neuropathic pain is relatively common in MS. Treatment is individualized and depends on the quality of pain, severity, and location. Some medications that may be useful include amitriptyline, nortriptyline, carbamazepine, gabapentin, and mexiletine. Nonsteroidal medication may be tried. Narcotic analgesics are occasionally necessary.

3. *Fatigue.* Frequent naps and energy conservation are helpful in MS-related fatigue. Make sure there are no nighttime sleep disorders complicating the course. Amantidine and modafinil have been shown to help fatigue in MS. Other agents that are used include methylphenidate (Ritalin) and other stimulant medications in selected patients.

4. *Tremor.* Drug therapy occasionally may be helpful, but typically the effects are short lived. Agents include isoniazid, benzodiazepines, primidone, and propranolol. Weighted bracelets are often the most practical approach. Surgical thalamotomy has been tried in some cases with reduction in tremor but often without significant functional improvement. Studies have shown that low doses of topiramate or levetiracetam may be useful in such tremor.

5. *Bladder and bowel dysfunction.* It has been shown that one cannot predict the mechanism of bladder dysfunction based on symptoms alone. Thus patients with troublesome bladder symptoms should be referred to a urologist for urodynamic testing. The most common pattern of bladder dysfunction in MS is detrusor-sphincter-dyssynergia (DSD). Detrusor muscle hyperreflexia can be managed with anticholinergic agents, including oxybutynin, propantheline, and imipramine. These drugs will decrease symptoms of frequency, nocturia, urgency, and incontinence, but one must guard against subsequent urinary retention and resultant urinary tract infection, especially because with DSD, the external sphincter does not relax appropriately. Monitoring for and treating urinary tract infections is important. Acidication of the urine with ascorbic acid (vitamin C) or cranberry juice may protect against gram-negative infections. Chronic antibiotic therapy may lead to resistant organisms. Often patients require intermittent self-catheterization to ensure complete bladder emptying. Indwelling catheteriza-

tion carries the risk of increased infection. Surgical procedures are sometimes necessary. Constipation is not uncommon in MS, especially in more severely affected, wheelchair-confined patients. Bowel urgency and incontinence are less common. Most patients benefit from increased fluid and roughage in their diet. Metamucil or glycerin suppositories are often helpful. Cathartics should be used only as a last resort.

6. *Sexual dysfunction.* Erectile dysfunction is common in patients with spinal cord involvement. Patients should be referred to a urologist. Approaches include sildenafil citrate, intracorporeal papaverine, phentolamine or prostaglandin injections, or at times penile prostheses.

Suggested Reading

Frohman EM. Multiple sclerosis. *Med Clin North Am* 2003;87(4):867–897.

Frohman E, Phillips T, Kokel K, et al. Disease-modifying therapy in multiple sclerosis: strategies for optimizing management. *Neurology* 2002; 8:227–236.

Kieseier BC, Hartung HP. Current disease-modifying therapies in multiple sclerosis. *Semin Neurol* 2003;23(2):133–146.

McDonald I, Compston A, Edan G, et al. Recommended diagnostic criteria for MS. *Ann Neurol* 2001;50:121–127.

Weiner HL. A 21 point hypothesis on the etiology and treatment of multiple sclerosis. *Can J Neurol Sci* 1998;25:93–101.

Weiner HL, Cohen JA. Treatment of multiple sclerosis with cyclophosphamide: critical review of clinical and immunologic effects. *Mult Scler* 2002;8(2):142–154.

Chapter 22

Neurology of Diabetes

Case

A 65-year-old woman with adult-onset diabetes presents with the recent onset of aching pain in both thighs, difficulty going up stairs, and a 40-pound weight loss. She has patchy sensory loss over the anterior thighs, absent knee and ankle jerks, and weakness of iliopsoas muscles and knee extensors. Her symptoms gradually improve after adding insulin to her oral agent and beginning a high-protein diet.

Diagnosis

Diabetic lumbar plexopathy.

Patients with diabetes frequently complain of neurologic symptoms; "neuropathy" is a classic diabetic complication. Most of the neurologic complications of diabetes involve the peripheral nervous system. Cerebrovascular disease and metabolic encephalopathies caused by hypoglycemia or hyperglycemia are the most common central nervous system complications of diabetes.

DIABETIC NEUROPATHY

Distal Polyneuropathy

Distal polyneuropathy is the most common diabetic neuropathy; it manifests as a slowly progressive, symmetric, distal ("glove and stocking"), predominantly sensory polyneuropathy. It is caused primarily by metabolic changes in the nerve with chronically elevated blood sugars. Ankle jerks are generally absent, and vibration sense is diminished; pin and temperature may be decreased distally in the legs more than the arms. This benign neuropathy usually does not bring the patient to the physician unless there are burning dysesthesias ("burning foot" neuropathy), which are caused by small fiber involvement. The loss of sensation can lead to trophic changes and injury from trauma, infection, ulceration, and joint destruction.

Mononeuropathy

Mononeuropathy is a dramatic diabetic neuropathy that probably results from nerve infarction. The onset of motor and sensory loss in one nerve is abrupt and often painful; the involved nerve may be tender. Prognosis is good, and recovery usually occurs in 4 to 6 months. Treatment is with physical therapy and appropriate support (splints where needed). There is a predilection for certain nerves. The most commonly affected are as follows:

1. *Oculomotor (III) nerve.* The patient has diplopia and may have pain over the eye. There is an almost total ophthalmoplegia. (Lateral eye movement is spared.) The pupillary fibers are on the outer perimeter of the nerve, and vascular infarction occurs centrally. Thus, the pupil is of normal size and reacts to light. It is not large and unreactive as in other third nerve palsies (e.g., those caused by compression). *Remember, the clue to a "diabetic third" is that the pupillary fibers usually are spared.*
2. *Abducens (VI) nerve.* There is an isolated inability to move the eye laterally. Remember, a sixth nerve palsy also may be the first sign of increased intracranial pressure. (Check for headache and papilledema.)
3. *Femoral nerve.* There is pain in the lateral and anterior thigh, weakness and atrophy of quadriceps (extension at knee) plus weakness of iliopsoas (flexion of hip), and a diminished or absent knee jerk (see Chapter 10).
4. *Radial nerve and peroneal nerve.* There is wristdrop or footdrop, respectively (see Chapter 10).
5. *Facial (VII) nerve.* Bell's palsy is more common in diabetics (see Chapter 10).

Entrapment Neuropathy

Entrapment neuropathies such as median nerve at the wrist and ulnar nerve at the elbow are more common in patients with diabetes. Carpal tunnel release may be helpful even in the presence of diabetic neuropathy if focal entrapment is present.

Radiculopathy

Radiculopathy is secondary to involvement of the posterior root outside the spinal cord before it becomes a mixed nerve. Clinically, the patient complains of shooting pains, often confined to a single dermatome. This neuropathy may be difficult to distinguish from disc disease and fortunately resolves spontaneously. Lumbar and thoracic roots most frequently are affected, and involvement may be bilateral. Sometimes there is posterior column degeneration, resulting in posterior column dysfunction and shooting pains. If the patient has these symptoms plus an irregular pupil that accommodates but reacts poorly to light (sometimes seen in people with diabetes), the term "diabetic pseudotabes" is used.

Thoraco-Abdominal Radiculopathy

An important and clinically underappreciated neuropathy is diabetic *thoraco-abdominal radiculopathy*. In this condition multiple nerve roots are affected, causing a "sunburn" sensation over the abdomen or chest, commonly with focal bulging of the abdominal wall caused by associated muscle weakness. It may present early in diabetes and often is followed by an extensive gastrointestinal and surgical workup before the correct diagnosis is made. Careful sensory and reflex examination shows patchy sensory loss over the abdomen and chest, absent superficial abdominal reflexes, and a lax abdominal musculature. This neuropathy usually improves over several months with control of the diabetes.

Lumbar Plexopathy

Lumbar plexopathy generally is seen in older patients and consists of pain in the thighs and proximal muscle weakness and wasting, often of sudden onset. Notable features include increased pain at night and significant weight loss accompanying the onset. Quadriceps and hamstrings also may be weak, and the patient complains of myalgia and dysesthesias in the thighs. Knee and ankle reflexes are usually absent. There is evidence to indicate a microvascular ischemic process, with proximal motor nerves of the lower extremities being affected preferentially. The prognosis is good, with recovery occurring over 6 to 12 months, particularly with optimum control of the diabetes and improved protein intake. Check for other causes of proximal muscle weakness (e.g., endocrine myopathy or polymyositis).

Autonomic Neuropathy

The most common manifestations of *autonomic neuropathy* are orthostatic hypotension (treat with elastic stockings, mineralocorticoids, midodrine, etc.), nocturnal diarrhea, impotence, urinary retention, and abdominal distension. Autonomic neuropathy explains various late problems in diabetes, including silent myocardial ischemia or infarction; loss of "autonomic" symptoms of hypoglycemia; and small, poorly reactive pupils to light with preserved accommodation. Early satiety ("filling up" with small amounts of food), gustatory sweating (profuse sweating only in the face and upper body after a meal), nocturnal diarrhea, and loss of distal limb sweating are other common manifestations of this entity.

COMMENTS ABOUT DIABETES AND THE NERVOUS SYSTEM

1. The physician should make sure that the neuropathies are associated with diabetes and do not represent symptoms caused by other treatable processes.
2. Support and physical therapy are important during the period of recovery. Meticulous foot care is vital in preventing ulcers and other complications of peripheral neuropathy.
3. There is evidence that neuropathies may be prevented or ameliorated by careful blood sugar control in the patient with diabetes and that insulin is often more effective than oral agents.
4. Drugs such as amitriptyline, phenytoin, carbamazepine, gabapentin, lamotrigine, or nonsteroidal antiinflammatory agents may be useful for the pain or paresthesias of diabetic neuropathy. Capsaicin ointment, a topical ointment made from an extract of chili peppers, is effective in some patients.
5. Other helpful measures include frequently examining the feet for ulcers or infection; wearing comfortable, well-fitting

shoes; and avoiding other toxins, such as alcohol, to prevent additive neuropathies.

6. Workup of suspected diabetic neuropathy should include assessing duration and control of diabetes and checking for foot deformities and skin changes. Electromyogram and nerve conduction studies are often helpful in differential diagnosis.

7. Cerebrospinal fluid protein frequently is elevated in diabetes but rarely exceeds 100 mg/dL because of diabetes alone.

8. It has been reported that some diabetic neuropathies may be treated with antiinflammatory medication or autoimmune therapy.

9. The restless leg syndrome is a common early manifestation of diabetic neuropathy. It may be treated with anti-parkinsonian medications, such as carbidopa-levodopa or pramipexole, for symptomatic relief.

Central Nervous System Disorders Associated with Diabetes

1. *Diabetic coma* and *hypoglycemia* are common, particularly in patients with insulin-dependent diabetes. Remember to draw blood to test the blood sugar level and administer 50% glucose intravenously to all patients presenting with coma of uncertain cause.

2. Patients with hypoglycemia may present with behavioral disturbances, seizures, and focal neurologic deficits that clear after glucose administration.

3. Treatment of *hyperglycemia* and coma may result in hypokalemia and a flaccid paralysis.

4. Cerebral edema may occur in both diabetic ketoacidosis and in nonketotic hyperglycemic states.

5. Occasionally, patients with diabetes with highly elevated sugars (e.g., hyperosmotic nonketotic states) will have continuous focal motor seizure activity that resists treatment until the glucose is controlled (epilepsia partialis continua).

6. Patients with diabetes are at increased risk for cerebrovascular disease, with both large- and small-vessel atherosclerosis.

7. *Cervical spondylosis* is more apt to be symptomatic in the patient with diabetes. There may be hyperactive reflexes at the knees with up-going toes (secondary to compression of the cord at the cervical region), loss of ankle jerks and vibra-

tion sense (secondary to compression of the cord at the cervical region), and loss of ankle jerks and vibration sense (secondary to the diabetic neuropathy).

Suggested Reading

Asbury AK. Understanding diabetic neuropathy. *N Engl J Med* 1988;319: 577–581.

Barohn RJ, Sahenk Z, Warmolts JR, et al. The Bruns-Garland syndrome (Diabetic Amyotrophy) revisited 100 years later. *Arch Neurol* 1991;48: 1130–1135.

Cohen J, Gross K. Autonomic neuropathy: clinical presentation and differential diagnosis. *Geriatrics* 1990;45:33–42.

Giugliano D, Marfella R, Quatraro A, et al. Tolrestat for mild diabetic neuropathy. *Ann Intern Med* 1993;118:7–11.

Greene DA. Diabetic neuropathy. *Ann Rev Med* 1990;41:303–317.

Harati Y. Diabetic peripheral neuropathy. *Ann Int Med* 1987;107:546–559.

Harati Y. Diabetes and the nervous system. *Endocrinol Metab Clin North Am* 1996;25(2):325–359.

Harati Y, Niakan E. Diabetic thoracoabdominal neuropathy; a cause for chest and abdominal pain. *Arch Intern Med* 1986;146:1493–1494.

Krendel DA, Costigan DA, Hopkins LC. Successful treatment of neuropathies in patients with diabetes mellitus. *Arch Neurol* 1995;52: 1053–1061.

McCall AL. Diabetes mellitus and the central nervous system. *Int Rev Neurobiol* 2002;51:415–453.

Pourmand R. Diabetic neuropathy. *Neurol Clin* 1997;15:569–576.

Watkins PJ, Thomas PK. Diabetes mellitus and the nervous system. *J Neurol Neurosurg Psychiat* 1998;65(5):620–632.

Wein TH, Albers JW. Diabetic neuropathies. *Phys Med Rehab Clin North Am* 2001;12(2):307–320.

Chapter 23

Malignancy and the Nervous System

Case

A varsity soccer player falls down on the field and has clonic shaking of his right arm that lasts for 10 minutes. He is brought to the emergency room, where examination shows a right facial droop, drift of the right arm, bilateral papilledema, and a slightly flat affect. He has been having worsening morning headache for 3 weeks. Brain magnetic resonance imaging (MRI) shows an irregularly enhancing mass lesion in the left temporal lobe with extensive edema.

Diagnosis

Probable glioblastoma multiforme, left temporal lobe.

Malignancy may affect the nervous system in two ways: (a) direct involvement by primary or metastatic brain or spinal cord tumor; and (b) by nonmetastatic effects, when nervous system dysfunction is associated with malignancy elsewhere in the body. The prevalence of neurologic complications of cancer is increasing with improvement of treatment and increased longevity in patients with cancer.

SIGNS AND SYMPTOMS OF BRAIN TUMOR

These signs and symptoms apply to primary and metastatic central nervous system (CNS) tumors.

1. Does the patient have *headache*? Headache is one of the most common symptoms, present in approximately two thirds of patients. It often occurs in the morning, when intracranial pressure is higher.
2. Other signs and symptoms include seizures, personality changes, hemiplegia, and visual disturbances. Mental changes, especially memory loss and decreased alertness, are often important subtle clues of intracranial tumor.
3. Patients often have a *gait disturbance.*
4. *Seizures* associated with tumor are characteristically focal. They may be Jacksonian—a focal seizure that begins in one extremity then "marches" until it becomes a generalized convulsion. New-onset seizures in a middle-aged adult often are caused by a brain tumor.
5. Check for *papilledema* or sixth nerve paresis caused by increased intracranial pressure.
6. Sometimes there may be bleeding within a tumor or vessel occlusion, creating the clinical picture of a stroke. Some tumors have a propensity to bleed (e.g., melanoma, hypernephroma, choriocarcinoma).

PRIMARY BRAIN TUMORS

Primary brain tumors, although uncommon, are a significant cause of death in middle-aged adults. The most common types are glioblastoma multiforme, astrocytoma, meningioma, and pituitary adenoma. Primary CNS lymphoma is becoming more common, particularly in patients with acquired immune deficiency syndrome (AIDS).

Glioblastoma

Glioblastoma comprises 20% of all intracranial tumors. It usually is located in the hemispheres in adults, with peak incidence in middle age. It may present with headache, seizure, or a personality change. It is a neoplasm of astrocytic-type cells and is a vascular tumor with irregular enhancement on MRI and computed tomography (CT). Irrespective of treatment, it carries a poor prognosis for long-term survival. Because the margins are not well defined, it is usually not a "surgically curable" tumor. Radiation therapy and resection may slow the progression temporarily.

Newer radiotherapy techniques have included radioactive implants, stereotactic radiosurgery (linear accelerator or gamma knife), charged and heavy particles, radiation with radiosensitizers, hyperthermia, and boron neutron capture therapy. To date, none of these techniques have proved to be superior to standard radiotherapy.

Astrocytoma

Astrocytoma is a slow-growing astrocytic tumor with a better long-term prognosis, but cure is rare. Astrocytoma may form large cavities. In approximately half of patients, it presents with seizures. The role of early radiation is disputed, but surgical treatment is common in moderate-grade tumors. The treatment of low-grade astrocytomas remains controversial. Other, less common primary tumors of the brain include oligodendrogliomas, medulloblastomas, and teratomas.

Meningioma

Meningioma is a benign tumor of the dura, located over the surface of the brain (convexity, wing of the sphenoid, skull base) in the spinal canal as an intradural/extramedullary lesion and rarely in an intraventricular location. It is more common in women and in the elderly. Thoracic spinal meningioma occurs particularly in elderly women. Meningiomas enhance on MRI and CT, and angiography shows a tumor blush. Surgical resection of this tumor is usually curative unless only partial removal is possible or anaplastic pathology is present. Certain meningiomas that are benign cannot be completely resected because of their location such as in the cavernous sinus or growing into the sagittal sinus.

Pituitary Adenoma

Pituitary adenoma is an endocrine tumor that may cause amenorrhea, acromegaly, Cushing's disease, or rarely hyperthyroidism. It may be nonsecreting, causing symptoms by pressure on the optic chiasm and normal pituitary gland. Classically, it causes a bitemporal hemianopsia (loss of temporal fields of vision) because of compression of the nasal retinal fibers passing through the chiasm. Treatment is surgical or medical with dopamine agonists such as bromocriptine. Other treatment modalities include radiotherapy and endocrine replacement therapy.

Primary Central Nervous System Lymphoma

Primary CNS lymphoma is a B-cell tumor with a periventricular localization that may involve the eye in 20% of cases. (Vitreous biopsy may be diagnostic.) It is becoming more frequent and is common in patients with AIDS. It is often deep in the brain and usually multicentric. It is rapidly progressive and treated by stereotactic biopsy, radiation, steroids, and chemotherapy. It is usually unresectable. In patients infected with the human immunodeficiency virus, it may be difficult to distinguish lymphoma from toxoplasmosis; stereotactic biopsy may be helpful. Prognosis is poor when AIDS is present. Because steroid therapy may lyse CNS lymphoma, delay use of steroids until after biopsy if CNS lymphoma is suspected. A multidrug chemotherapy combination including methotrexate, procarbazine, vincristine, dexamethasone, and cytarabine plus radiation therapy has been shown to produce an increase in median survival of 41 months, compared with 10 months for patients receiving radiotherapy alone. Newer regimens of high-dose methotrexate also have been used.

INTRACRANIAL METASTASES

Which Tumors Invade the Brain?

Up to 25% of patients with cancer have cerebral metastases at autopsy. Metastatic tumor reaches the brain through hematogenous spread and generally after first invading the lung. This accounts for the high incidence of intracranial metastases with *lung* and *breast* tumors. Tumors of the gastrointestinal tract may metastasize to the brain, although they do so less frequently and generally invade the liver and lung first. *Hypernephroma* and *melanoma* are important sources of CNS metastases but are less common tumors. *Prostatic* carcinoma, a common tumor in elderly men, rarely metastasizes to the brain. Tumors of the *cervix* and *ovary* also metastasize to the brain infrequently.

When Do Tumors Metastasize to the Brain?

Most metastases occur within 2 years of discovery of the primary lesion, although they sometimes can appear years after the removal of a primary source (e.g., with kidney or breast cancer). Conversely, a metastatic tumor may be the first sign of a primary neoplasm elsewhere, especially with lung cancer.

When a neurologic symptom (e.g., seizure) is secondary to a brain metastasis, obvious neurologic progression usually will occur within 6 months. For example, a patient with known breast carcinoma who has a convulsion and then remains neurologically intact for 6 months probably did not experience the seizure because of a cerebral metastasis.

LABORATORY INVESTIGATION

1. MRI with gadolinium enhancement is the most sensitive test for detection of brain tumor, especially in the posterior fossa. Contrast-enhanced CT is also accurate. Contrast-enhanced MRI is particularly useful if leptomeningeal metastases are suspected. Electroencephalogram (EEG) is not a good screening tool for tumor, although it is often abnormal and may be helpful to detect seizure activity related to tumor. A lumbar puncture (LP) should not be performed if an intracranial tumor is suspected because the LP may cause herniation if mass effect is present (see Chapter 30).
2. Arteriography is rarely necessary for diagnosis, although it may help distinguish primary from metastatic lesions. Arteriography may be helpful before surgery on a meningioma to delineate the vascular supply of the tumor.
3. There is increasing use of stereotactic brain biopsy as a method of establishing the correct diagnosis with low morbidity, particularly for lesions that are not considered resectable. However, pathologic diagnosis sometimes may be difficult because of the small amount of tissue obtained with this kind of biopsy.
4. The physician must evaluate each patient individually in terms of which studies to perform.

TREATMENT

The treatment of *primary brain tumor* depends on the tumor type and location. Meningiomas are usually surgically removable.

Low-grade astrocytomas and oligodendrogliomas are best treated by surgery plus irradiation. High-grade astrocytomas (glioblastoma multiforme) are treated by resection plus irradiation or, depending on location, partial removal plus irradiation. There is increasing use of chemotherapy—such as 1,3-bis-(2 chloroethyl) 1-nitrosouria (BCNU) intravenously or as Gliadel wafers (Rhûne-Poulenc-Rorer, Collegeville, PA) implanted at the time of resection—which prolongs survival. Chemotherapy trials are available for most patients with primary brain tumor. Tumors showing symptomatic mass effect may be treated with dexamethasone.

In patients with *metastatic brain tumor,* one first must determine whether the brain is involved by single or multiple metastases; MRI with gadolinium is the most sensitive test. Documented *multiple metastases* are treated with steroids and whole brain irradiation. Symptoms are ameliorated with steroids to reduce cerebral edema. One randomized study showed similar efficacy using 1 mg qid and 4 mg qid, with a reduced side effect profile in the low-dose regimen. Higher doses are used for impending herniation. Irradiation improves length and quality of survival. Chemotherapy may be added. Treatment of a *single metastasis* is surgical if the patient is a good operative candidate and the lesion is surgically accessible. In addition to offering palliation, other disease processes sometimes are found at operation (e.g., subdural hematoma, brain abscess, primary brain tumor). Radiosurgery provides another approach to single metastases less than 3 cm in diameter.

METASTATIC TUMOR TO THE SPINAL CORD

Management

Metastatic tumor to the cord (generally epidural implant) may compress the cord; it constitutes a neurologic emergency (see Chapter 9). Carcinoma of the lung, breast, or prostate or lymphomas and leukemias may cause spinal cord compression. Back pain, tenderness, change in urinary frequency, or symptoms of root involvement often appear before compression. Plain films of the spine usually are abnormal, but the findings may be subtle. Thus, MRI or bone scan is often helpful. See Chapter 9 for evaluation and treatment of acute spinal cord compression.

LEUKEMIA AND LYMPHOMA

Leukemia and lymphoma are malignant processes frequently associated with nervous system dysfunction and may invade the brain and spinal cord. With more effective treatment and with patients living longer, there has been an increasing incidence of CNS complications.

Leukemia

Leukemia is associated with a triad of neurologic complications.

1. *Intracranial hemorrhage* is common in leukemia and usually is related to a low platelet count or a high leukocyte count (more than 100,000/mm). Intracranial bleeding occurs in multiple areas (not usually one, as in hypertensive bleeding) and often is associated with systemic bleeding. Once bleeding has occurred, transfusion therapy is usually of little benefit.

2. Leukemic infiltration of meninges (of brain and spinal cord) and nerve roots is common and frequently occurs when the patient is in hematologic remission. Meningeal leukemia usually presents as headache, nausea, and vomiting secondary to increased intracranial pressure (there may be papilledema); seizures, visual disturbances, and ataxia also occur. Cranial nerve palsies occur (commonly III, VI, and VII). *Diagnosis* is made by LP. Look for elevated pressure, leukemic cells, elevated protein, and decreased sugar. MRI with gadolinium may detect leukemic infiltration and is particularly useful in detecting leptomeningeal spread. Treatment with intrathecal methotrexate and radiotherapy is usually effective and may be given prophylactically to patients with leukemia in hematologic remission, before CNS complications occur.

   Note: The hypothalamic–pituitary axis may be involved, resulting in hyperphagia (weight gain) or diabetes insipidus. In addition, there may be infiltration surrounding cord and roots; look for signs and symptoms of cord compression or root dysfunction.

3. *Infection.* These patients are prone to CNS infection, usually bacterial (e.g., *Listeria*) and fungal (e.g., *Cryptococcus*). Whenever CNS symptoms are present, even if they are only drowsi-

ness and headache, perform an LP to look for meningeal leukemia or infection, after excluding a mass lesion by CT scan or MRI.

Note: Herpes zoster is common, at times affecting roots with prior leukemic infiltration.

Lymphoma

Patients with *lymphoma* are subject to the same complications as those with leukemia, except for intracerebral hemorrhage. Leptomeningeal spread is common in non-Hodgkin's lymphoma.

Spinal cord compression by lymphoma is especially common, as are compressive syndromes in other parts of the nervous system: brachial plexus, recurrent laryngeal nerve (vocal cord paralysis), phrenic nerve, cervical sympathetics (Horner's syndrome), and lumbosacral roots. Treatment of choice is radiation and chemotherapy. The compressive syndromes are more common in lymphomas than in leukemias, unlike primary CNS lymphoma. Systemic lymphoma rarely causes an intracranial mass lesion, although it has been reported with reticulum cell sarcoma (histiocytic lymphoma).

Note: Meningeal involvement by tumors other than lymphoma and leukemia (*carcinomatous meningitis*) occurs most commonly with breast cancer. As with meningeal leukemia (see earlier), look for symptoms of increased intracranial pressure, multiple cranial nerve palsies, radiculopathy, and cerebrospinal fluid (CSF) abnormalities (malignant cells and high protein). Treatment consists of intrathecal chemotherapy and radiotherapy. A reservoir for injecting the drug(s) often is used.

NONMETASTATIC COMPLICATIONS OF MALIGNANCY

Paraneoplastic Syndromes

Paraneoplastic syndromes are a unique group of symptoms that reflects the remote effects of malignancy on the nervous system. The etiology of these distant effects varies and may be related to immunologic, hormonal, or toxic factors elaborated by the tumor.

A variety of unique neurologic syndromes may be the first manifestation of a malignancy elsewhere. Distant neurologic dysfunction as a result of malignancy is known as a paraneoplastic syndrome. Symptoms associated with these syndromes sometimes disappear when the primary tumor is removed. Certain neoplasms such as small-cell lung cancer are more commonly associated with neurologic findings.

Cerebellar Degeneration

With cerebellar degeneration, there is unsteadiness in gait and difficulty using limbs, progressing to slurred speech and trouble eating. Symptoms usually progress over weeks. Nystagmus is often not present. Cerebellar degeneration has been reported primarily with tumors of the lung, ovary, and breast. Although the cerebellar dysfunction is most striking, there may be other evidence of associated CNS dysfunction, including mental changes, muscle weakness, peripheral neuropathy, and extensor plantar responses. Anti-Purkinje cell antibodies have been detected in the serum and CSF of some of these patients, and patients with such antibodies have a more rapid course.

Myasthenic (Eaton-Lambert) Syndrome

Myasthenic (Eaton-Lambert) syndrome most frequently is associated with bronchial carcinoma in men. It presents as a generalized proximal weakness and easy fatigability. Associated features include dry mouth, impotence, and peripheral paresthesias. Trouble with eye movements or difficulty swallowing is less common. The characteristic feature of this syndrome is that a few muscle contractions must be carried out before full strength is reached, after which the patient fatigues (in myasthenia gravis, full strength is present at the outset and diminishes with exercise). This can be demonstrated by electrodiagnostic studies. Eaton-Lambert is a presynaptic disorder of the neuromuscular junction, whereas myasthenia gravis affects the postsynaptic junction. Treatment with guanidine or aminopyridine (which facilitate acetylcholine release) is more beneficial than anticholinesterase medication. The myasthenic syndrome may occur in the absence of malignancy; this syndrome has an autoimmune basis. Patients with this syndrome may be abnormally sensitive to muscle relaxants used in anesthesia, at times with life-threatening respiratory suppression.

Sensory Neuropathy

There is numbness and tingling of the upper and lower extremities associated with a sensory ataxia. Reflexes are absent, and there may be proximal muscle wasting in the lower extremities. A sensorimotor neuropathy also has been associated with malignancy.

Opsoclonus-Myoclonus

Opsoclonus, a peculiar jerking of the eyes to and fro, and myoclonus, a sudden jerking of large muscle groups, may be seen as remote effects of cancer (neuroblastoma in children, various tumors in adults).

Dementia

Dementia rarely may be associated with malignancy (carcinoma of the lung), secondary to "limbic encephalitis," which causes severely impaired memory and altered behavior. There may be associated diffuse changes in the nervous system and a concomitant sensory neuropathy. The CSF is usually abnormal.

Polymyositis and Dermatomyositis

Both polymyositis and dermatomyositis are associated with neoplasm and may antedate the appearance of the tumor. Myositis presents as proximal muscle weakness. The muscles are usually not tender. If tumor eradication is impossible or does not help, steroids may be of benefit. Remember, the importance of these remote effects of malignancy is the clue they offer that a malignancy is present, although they may appear when the tumor is well established. A characteristic feature of these syndromes is that they are seldom "pure"; they spill over to involve more than one area of the nervous system.

Metabolic Encephalopathy

Patients with cancer are prone to develop lethargy, confusion, and behavior disturbances as the result of metabolic abnormalities related to, but not directly resulting from, the underlying cancer. Examples include uremia; hepatic and respiratory failure; electrolyte disturbances such as hypercalcemia, hyponatremia, and hypoglycemia; and drug overdoses. Patients with cancer also are prone to develop infections of various types, and sepsis may cause a metabolic encephalopathy. Metabolic brain disease is suggested by lethargy, clouding of consciousness, a fluctuating picture, myoclonus, a lack of focal signs, and confirmatory laboratory studies such as a normal CT scan or MRI and an abnormal EEG that shows bilateral slowing without focal features.

Vascular Disorders

Patients with cancer are prone to develop vascular disorders, such as cerebral infarction secondary to disseminated intravascular coagulation, and hypercoagulable states, venous sinus thromboses, or emboli from nonbacterial endocarditis (marantic endocarditis). They also are prone to intracerebral, subarachnoid, or subdural hemorrhage caused by thrombocytopenia or other coagulation disorder. Sometimes thrombosis in patients with cancer may not respond to treatment with warfarin and require subcutaneous heparin.

Bone Marrow Transplantation

Bone marrow transplantation (BMT) carries several risks: toxicity from chemotherapy, infection caused by immune suppression, bleeding related to thrombocytopenia, and graft versus host disease. More than half the patients undergoing BMT develop neurologic dysfunction. The most common neurologic side effect is a metabolic encephalopathy. CNS bacterial, viral, or fungal infection may occur as a result of profound immunosuppression (e.g., cytomegalovirus encephalitis, herpes zoster radiculitis). There may be thrombotic infarction or hemorrhage. Other neurologic syndromes such as mononeuritis multiplex, transverse myelitis, and myositis may be related to graft versus host disease. In children, cerebral atrophy, neuropsychologic dysfunction, and leukoencephalopathy also have been reported following BMT.

Other

Cancer patients may develop side effects of therapy, such as radiation myelopathy and neuropathy or encephalopathy or peripheral neuropathy secondary to chemotherapeutic agents (especially vincristine and cisplatinum). *Progressive multifocal leukoencephalopathy* usually is seen in patients with a compromised immune system. This occurs in patients with malignancies such as lymphomas or secondary to immunosuppression from chemotherapy or AIDS. Clinically, patients develop rapidly progressive deterioration of mental state and multiple focal neurologic deficits with multifocal white matter lesions with progression over a period of 6 months to 2 years. The clinical picture may be confused with multiple strokes. It is caused by a papovavirus that infects oligodendrocytes and astrocytes.

Suggested Reading

Alexander E. Recurrent brain metastases. *Neurosurg Clin North Am* 1996;7:517–526.

Balm M, Hammack J. Leptomeningeal carcinomatosis. *Arch Neurol* 1996;53:626–632.

Black PM. Brain tumors. *N Engl J Med* 1991;324:1471–1476, 1555–1564.

Brem H, Piantadosi S, Burger PC, et al. Placebo-controlled trial of safety and efficacy of intraoperative controlled delivery by biodegradable polymers of chemotherapy for recurrent gliomas. *Lancet* 1995;345: 1008–1012.

Byrne TN. Spinal cord compression from epidural metastases. *N Engl J Med* 1992:327:614–619.

Cher L, Glass J, Harsh GR, et al. Therapy of primary CNS lymphoma with methotrexate-based chemotherapy and deferred radiotherapy. *Neurology* 1996;46:1757–1759.

Clouston PD, DeAngelis LM, Posner JB. The spectrum of neurological disease in patients with systemic cancer. *Ann Neurol* 1992:31:268–273.

Constine LS, Woolf PD, Cann D, et al. Hypothalamic-pituitary dysfunction after radiation for brain tumors. *N Engl J Med* 1993;328:87–94.

Freilich RJ, Delattre JY, Monjour A, et al. Chemotherapy without radiation therapy as initial treatment of primary CNS lymphoma in older patients. *Neurology* 1996;46:435–439.

Jackson AC. Acute viral infections. *Curr Opin Neurol* 1995;8:170–174.

Li B, Yu J, Suntharalingam M. Comparison of three treatment options for single brain metastasis from lung cancer. *Int J Cancer* 2000;90:37–45.

Patchell RA, Tibbs PA, Walsh JW, et al. A randomized trial of surgery in the treatment of single metastases to the brain. *N Engl J Med* 1990:322:494–500.

Posner JB. *Neurologic complications of cancer.* Philadelphia: FA Davis, 1995.

Posner JB. Paraneoplastic syndromes. *Curr Opin Neurol* 1997;10:471–476.

Rees J. Neurological manifestations of malignant disease. *Hosp Med* 2000;61(9):319–325.

Rogers LR. Cerebrovascular complications in cancer patients. *Oncology* 1994;8:23–30.

Steck AJ. Neurological manifestations of malignant and non-malignant dysglobulinaemias. *J Neurol* 1998;245;624–639.

Vecht CJ, Hovestadt A, Verbiest H, et al. Dose-effect relationship of dexamethasone on Karnofsky performance in metastatic brain tumors: a randomized study of doses of 4,8, and 16 mg per day. *Neurology* 1994;44:675–680.

Weller M, Schmidt C, Roth W, et al. Chemotherapy of human malignant glioma: prevention of efficacy by dexamethasone? *Neurology* 1997;48: 1704–1709.

Chapter 24

Central Nervous System Infections

Central nervous system (CNS) infections are suggested by a constellation of signs, symptoms, and laboratory studies. It is beyond the scope of this manual to discuss each CNS infection individually. This chapter aims to alert the house officer to consider CNS infection as a diagnostic possibility when certain clinical features coexist, to pursue a definitive diagnosis, and to institute appropriate treatment. The major groups of CNS infections include bacterial meningitis, viral meningitis, chronic meningitis, acute encephalitis, and brain abscess. See Chapter 25 for the treatment of acquired immune deficiency virus (AIDS)-related CNS infections.

HISTORY

The diagnosis of *meningitis* (inflammation of the meninges) is suggested when history includes the following:

- Fever
- Headache
- Stiff neck

Acute bacterial meningitis is a neurologic emergency, with symptoms developing over hours or days. Delay in diagnosis and treatment can lead to permanent injury or death. *Viral meningitis* is suggested by the constellation of fever, headache, and stiff neck; the cerebrospinal fluid (CSF) features include a lymphocytic pleocytosis, normal sugar, and negative culture for bacteria. *Chronic meningitis* has a more indolent presentation and may be associated with cranial nerve palsies, cognitive changes, or strokelike events.

The diagnosis of encephalitis (evidence of brain parenchymal involvement) is suggested when the history includes the following:

- Mental status changes (ranging from confusion to coma)
- Seizures
- Focal neurologic signs such as paralysis

The diagnosis of *brain abscess* is suggested by the following:

- Headache
- Focal signs and focal seizures
- Signs of increased intracranial pressures

Fever is seen in approximately 50% of adults and up to 80% of children with brain abscess. Note that the presentation of these entities may overlap (e.g., " meningoencephalitis").

Pursue the following points in the history:

1. Has there been a recent respiratory or gastrointestinal infection?
2. Has the patient had a recent infectious illness that may progress to meningitis (e.g., otitis media leading to pneumococcal meningitis)? Has the patient had a positive reaction to purified protein derivative or known exposure to tuberculosis?
3. Has the patient been exposed to others with infectious illness (e.g., meningococcus or *Haemophilus influenzae*)?
4. Has there been recent travel to another state (e.g., exposure to mosquitoes causing arbovirus-associated encephalitis) or another country (cysticercosis in Central America)?
5. Has there been a subtle personality change and low-grade fever (e.g., in chronic meningitis such as *Cryptococcus*)?
6. What is the patient's occupation (e.g., painter exposed to *Cryptococcus* in pigeon droppings)?
7. Does an *underlying disease* predispose the patient to CNS infection?
   - Lymphoma, leukemia
   - Other malignancy
   - Renal failure
   - Human immunodeficiency virus (HIV)/AIDS and other immunodeficiency states

- Alcoholism
- Diabetes
- Posttransplant patient
- Asplenic (functional or surgical)

8. Is the patient receiving a drug(s) that predisposes to infection?
   - Chemotherapy
   - Immunosuppressant or immunomodulator
   - Corticosteroids
9. Has the patient had a recent illness such as mumps or chickenpox that may be followed by meningitis or meningoencephalitis?
10. Is the patient bacteremic, or has the patient recently been bacteremic? This increases the chances of secondary CNS infection?
11. Has there been a recent head injury?
12. Has there been a recent neurosurgical procedure or penetrating skull trauma?
13. Has there been a recent insect bite leading to Lyme disease or rickettsial infection, which mimics bacterial meningitis?

PHYSICAL AND NEUROLOGIC EXAMINATION

1. Check vital signs. Temperature may be higher in bacterial than in viral CNS infection. Herpes simplex encephalitis often results in a high fever (104° to 105°F). Tachycardia is seen in bacterial and viral CNS infection.
2. Check eardrums; examine sinuses for tenderness.
3. Check for stiff neck. Look for Kernig's sign (with thigh flexed on abdomen patient resists knee extension) or Brudzinski's sign (attempt to flex the neck results in reflex flexion of the knee and hip). Remember that the elderly, infants, and immunosuppressed patients may have meningitis without prominent meningeal signs. Comatose patients may not have meningismus.
4. Look for stigmata of chronic liver disease and chronic lung disease as a predisposing factor for CNS infection.
5. Look for peripheral signs of embolization in a patient suspected of having subacute bacterial endocarditis or staphylococcal septicemia.
6. Examine the heart carefully (e.g., changing murmur in subacute bacterial endocarditis with valvular disease as source of septic embolism).

7. Examine for lymph-node enlargement or splenomegaly. These signs may suggest a lymphoproliferative disorder, in which CNS infections commonly are seen.

8. Is there evidence of CSF rhinorrhea caused by a defect or fracture in the cribriform plate? (Check an unexplained nasal discharge for the presence of CSF glucose.) Is there otorrhea caused by a fracture in the petrous portion of the temporal bone?

9. Examine for petechial or purpuric lesions caused by meningococcemia or staphylococcal bacteremia.

LABORATORY

1. All patients suspected of having meningitis should have a lumbar puncture (LP) and treatment with antibiotics as soon as possible. Record the opening pressure. If focal neurologic symptoms or signs are present and brain abscess is a consideration, obtain a contrast-enhanced computed tomography (CT) or magnetic resonance imaging (MRI) scan first, but do not allow significant delay when there is a high likelihood of meningitis. If meningitis is a reasonable possibility and imaging is necessary, it may be appropriate to give IV antibiotics immediately. Blood cultures should be drawn before antibiotics are begun. See Chapter 30 for a discussion of CSF examination. In addition, note the following points regarding meningitis and encephalitis:

   a. CSF pressure is usually moderately elevated in bacterial meningitis (200 to 300 mm H_2O) and mildly elevated in viral meningitis or encephalitis.

   b. Cell count in untreated bacterial meningitis may range from 100 to $10,000/mm^3$ with a predominance of neutrophils; the fluid is usually cloudy. In viral meningitis, cell counts of 10 to $1,000/mm^3$ with a predominance of mononuclear cells are expected.

   c. CSF glucose is usually less than 40 mg/dL in bacterial or tuberculous meningitis (or less than 60% of simultaneously obtained blood glucose), whereas it is usually *normal* or only modestly reduced in viral meningitis or encephalitis.

   d. CSF protein usually is elevated higher than 100 mg/dL in bacterial meningitis, whereas a mild elevation (50 to 100 mg/dL) is expected in viral meningitis or encephalitis. A mild elevation also may be encountered in partially treated meningitis.

e. Elevated CSF lactate levels commonly are encountered in patients with meningitis following neurosurgical procedures.

f. Gram stain usually detects the causative organism in bacterial meningitis. India ink stain is helpful in diagnosing cryptococcal meningitis, as are CSF and serum cryptococcal antigens. Bacterial antigens can be detected in the spinal fluid by a variety of special techniques and may be helpful if the patient received antibiotic therapy before the LP.

2. Routine laboratory tests may offer clues. The white blood cell count is usually markedly elevated in bacterial meningitis and mildly elevated or normal in viral meningitis.

3. Check for hyponatremia caused by inappropriate antidiuretic hormone secretion as a complicating feature in a meningitis patient with increasing lethargy.

4. Chest radiograph may demonstrate a source of CNS infection (e.g., pneumonia or bronchiectasis).

5. The electroencephalogram may be normal or slightly slow in meningitis and encephalitis, but it often shows focal features in brain abscess and paroxysmal features in the temporal lobe in herpes simplex encephalitis.

6. CT and MRI scans are usually normal in uncomplicated meningitis but often are focally abnormal in herpes simplex encephalitis (temporal lobe). They may demonstrate complications of meningitis such as subdural fluid collections, hydrocephalus, or cerebral infarction.

7. In patients with suspected viral CNS infections, obtain a serum specimen acutely, and save to compare with convalescent sera for an increase in antibody titers (e.g., in mumps infection).

8. In suspected enterovirus CNS infection (Coxsackie, Echo), the virus often is detected in stool specimens. Mumps virus may be isolated from saliva, throat washings, or CSF.

9. Bacteremia is present in many patients with bacterial meningitis and should be detected by appropriate blood cultures.

10. Beware of coagulopathy in patients with fulminant meningitis (especially meningococcus).

11. Use PCR (polymerase chain reaction) to identify herpes simplex; other viruses and tuberculosis will hasten diagnosis.

TREATMENT

Bacterial Meningitis

The mainstay of treatment of bacterial meningitis is intravenous antibiotics (see Table 24.1). For suspected undiagnosed bacterial meningitis in adults, start ceftriaxone 2 g intravenously (IV) every 12 hours. If penicillin-resistant pneumococcus is a concern, vancomycin 1g IV every 12 hours should be administered until susceptibilities are available. If Listeria is a consideration (immunosuppressed individual), ampicillin 2 g IV every 4 hours should be added to the regimen. Appropriate dosing modifications for age and renal function need to be considered for all patients. For those with a severe allergy to beta lactam antibiotics, chloramphenicol may be prescribed. Remember, if an LP is delayed for any reason, consider giving empiric antibiotics before LP. Early treatment is crucial in these patients.

TABLE 24.1.   Antibiotics Used for Meningitis[a]

Organism	Appropriate Antibiotics
Streptococcus pneumoniae	Penicillin G (only when sensitivities demonstrate MIC <0.1 µg/mL), ceftriaxone, vancomycin, chloramphenicol
Neisseria meningitidis	Penicillin G, ceftriaxone, chloramphenicol
Haemophilus influenzae	Ceftriaxone or cefotaxime, chloramphenicol, ampicillin (only for beta-lactamase negative-isolates)
Staphylococcus aureus	Nafcillin ± rifampin or vancomycin
Listeria monocytogenes	Ampicillin, trimethoprim-sulfamethoxazole
Escherichia coli, Klebsiella	Cefotaxime, ceftriaxone, meropenem, aztreonam
Proteus	Ceftriaxone, meropenem
Pseudomonas	Ceftazidime and aminoglycoside, meropenem

MIC, minimal inhibitory concentrations.

[a]The final selection of antimicrobial medications should be based on careful review of microbiology results, patient drug allergies, and renal status.

Other measures include the following:

1. Patients with meningitis may develop cerebral swelling (edema). If this occurs, treatment with mannitol (0.25 to 0.50 g/kg) or dexamethasone (10 mg IV then 4 mg every 6 hours) may be given. Intubation and hyperventilation may be used to lower $PaCO_2$ to 25 to 30 mmHg as a temporary measure.

2. Seizures are common in meningitis and usually are treated with intravenous phenytoin or fos-phenytoin.

3. Fluid restriction to 1,200 to 1,500 mL/day may be needed to reduce brain swelling or to control the syndrome of inappropriate antidiuretic hormone.

4. Early use of dexamethasone 0.15mg/kg IV every 6 hours for 2 days in children and dexamethasone 10 mg IV q6h × 4 days in adults may reduce unfavorable outcomes in adults and children with bacterial meningitis. The benefits of dexamethasone in adults may be greatest in the settings of pneumococcal meningitis when the administration of steroids precedes the administration of antibiotics by at least 15 minutes. Gastrointestinal bleeding is uncommon when used with these protocols.

5. Standard infection-control precautions (gloves, handwashing, face/eye/mouth shield) and additional droplet precautions are essential for all cases of known or suspected meningitis.

6. Family members, medical personnel, and others with close contact to patients with meningococcal meningitis should receive prophylaxis with one of the following regimens: ciprofloxacin 500-mg single oral dose (adults only), rifampin 600 mg orally every 12 hours for 2 days, or ceftriaxone 250 mg intramuscularly (adult dosing; check for appropriate pediatric dosing).

Viral Meningitis/Encephalitis

1. Treatment of *viral meningitis* is supportive.

2. In cases of nonherpetic *viral encephalitis*, treatment is also supportive and directed at possible complications. For herpes simplex encephalitis, acyclovir has greatly improved morbidity and mortality. Usual dosage is 10 mg/kg every 8 hours IV, with vigorous hydration to avoid nephrotoxicity.

The diagnosis of herpes simplex virus (HSV) encephalitis is based on the detection of HSV by PCR of the CSF and characteristic clinical and radiographic findings.

3. Take meticulous care to promptly and completely dispose of needles and syringes, and precautions should be undertaken in handling stool specimens in those with enteroviral infection.

4. Isolate patients suspected of having measles, chickenpox, or rubella.

5. Treat fever with acetaminophen or aspirin. A cooling blanket may be helpful for extreme hyperthermia.

6. Treat seizures that accompany encephalitis.

7. The first cases of West Nile encephalitis in North America were reported in the summer of 1999. Since that time, the disease has become endemic in this area. West Nile virus is a member of the flavivirus family. Transmission to humans occurs following the bite of infected mosquitos and, in rare cases, following blood transfusion or organ transplantation from an infected source patient. Most infections are asymptomatic. However, some patients develop significant neurologic sequelae, including encephalitis (generally indistinguishable from other forms of arboviral encephalitis) and ascending flaccid paralysis similar to polio or Guillain-Barré syndrome. Diagnosis is based on serologic assessment of the blood or CSF. In symptomatic individuals, CSF generally demonstrates a lymphocytic pleocytosis and elevated protein. Treatment remains supportive.

Chronic Meningitis

Chronic meningitis presents with variable signs of meningeal irritation, cranial nerve dysfunction, and focal or global CNS dysfunction lasting 4 weeks or more. There is CSF pleocytosis, which may be caused by infectious or noninfectious processes (e.g., tuberculosis, fungus, hypersensitivity reaction, CNS tumor, chronic HIV, syphilis, and sarcoidosis). Treatment depends on the specific etiology found.

Brain Abscess

If brain abscess is a consideration, avoid LP until mass lesion has been excluded by CT or MRI. Aspiration or excision of brain abscesses, with appropriate antibiotic coverage and steroid therapy for edema, is the usual treatment. More conservative management of small abscesses with empiric antibiotics and close radiologic follow-up is being used.

OTHER CNS INFECTIONS

Lyme Disease

Lyme disease is a tick-borne spirochetal infection (caused by Borrelia species) with systemic and nervous system manifestations. Neurologic complications of early Lyme disease include aseptic meningitis, cranial nerve palsies (especially facial nerve), mononeuritis multiplex, Guillain-Barré syndrome, and a painful radiculoneuropathy; late stage or chronic sequelae include sensory neuropathy, and, in rare cases, a chronic encephalopathy. Diagnosis may be difficult, and serology leads to overdiagnosis in endemic areas. [See Halperin (1996) for guidelines on diagnosis.] Patients with CNS complications of Lyme should have detectable antibodies in the serum and CSF; the absence of antibodies makes the diagnosis highly unlikely. Intravenous ceftriaxone (doses of 2 g/day for 2 to 4 weeks) is the therapy of choice for most neurologic complications of Lyme disease. Isolated facial nerve palsy, however, will respond adequately to oral doxycycline (if there is no evidence of CSF pleocytosis). Consider Lyme disease in a patient who has an unexplained meningitis, an unusual radiculopathy, Guillain-Barré syndrome, or an atypical facial palsy, especially when the typical rash or other key epidemiologic features (e.g., endemic area, tick bite) are present.

Repeated use of prolonged courses of antibiotics for so-called "chronic nervous system Lyme disease" has not been shown to improve long-term outcome in patients. Once a standard appropriate form of antibiotics has been used in patients with serologic evidence of Lyme disease, there is no justification for repeated treatments. Patients with multiple sclerosis may be misidentified as having CNS Lyme disease, particularly when such patients live in endemic areas.

Neurosyphilis

Syphilis is associated with multiple neurologic complications. Invasion of the CNS during early syphilis may be associated with acute *meningitis* but is often asymptomatic. In the absence of therapy, subacute or chronic meningitis may develop, accompanied by headache, cranial nerve palsies, seizures, and symptoms of increased intracranial pressure. In *meningovascular syphilis,* strokes caused by vessel invasion occur. In *tabes dorsalis,* there is inflammation of the dorsal roots and dorsal columns of the spinal cord, causing a sensory ataxia; bowel and bladder dysfunction; destruction of deafferented joints ("Charcot joints"); and episodes of severe, lancinating pains in the legs and body ("lightening pains"). Pupils are small, irregular, and reactive to accommodation but not to light ("Argyll-Robertson pupils"), probably because of a partial third-nerve injury. *General paresis* is a late manifestation of untreated syphilis with mental deterioration and occasional florid delusional ideas. Diagnosis is suggested by positive serologies [rapid plasma reagin (RPR) test or Venereal Disease Research Laboratory (VDRL) test] and confirmed by fluorescent treponemal antibody-absorption test (FTA-ABS) and an abnormal CSF. Treatment with penicillin is usually curative but may not reverse neurologic deficits.

Suggested Reading

DeGans J, van der Beek D. Dexamethasone in adults with bacterial meningitis. *N Engl J Med* 2002;347:1549–1556.

Halperin JJ, Logigian EL, Finkel MF, et al. Practice parameters for the diagnosis of patients with nervous system Lyme borreliosis. *Neurology* 1996;46:619–627.

Kanter MC, Hart RG. Neurologic complications of infective endocarditis. *Neurology* 1991;41:1015–1020.

Karlsson M, Hammers-Berggren S, Lindquist L, et al. Comparison of intravenous penicillin G and oral doxycycline for treatment of Lyme neuroborreliosis. *Neurology* 1994;44:1203–1207.

Kox LFF, Kuijper S, Kolk AHJ. Early diagnosis of tuberculous meningitis by polymerase chain reaction. *Neurology* 1995;45:2228–2232.

Jeffrey KJM, Read SJ, Mayon-White RT, et al. Diagnosis of viral infections of the central nervous system: clinical interpretation of PCR results. *Lancet* 1997;349:313–317.

Leib SL, Boscacci R, Gratzl O, et al. Predictive value of cerebrospinal fluid (CSF) lactate level versus CSF/blood glucose ratio for the diagnosis of bacterial meningitis following neurosurgery. *Clin Infect Dis* 1999;29:69–74.

Marra CM. Neurosyphilis: a guide for clinicians. *The Neurologist* 1995;1:157–166.

Quagliarello VJ, Scheld WM. Treatment of bacterial meningitis. *N Engl J Med* 1997;336:708–716.

Rosen SE. Shingles. *JAMA* 1993;269:1836–1839.

Steere AC, Taylor E, McHugh GL, Logigian EL. The overdiagnosis of Lyme disease. *JAMA* 1993;269:1812–1816.

Whitley RJ. Viral encephalitis. *N Engl J Med* 1990;323:242–250.

Chapter 25

AIDS and the Nervous System

Case

A 45-year-old man was exposed to the human immunodeficiency virus (HIV) by sharing an infected syringe for his heroin habit. He is admitted to the hospital with a progressive right-sided headache, a mild left hemiparesis, and a flat affect. His brain magnetic resonance imaging (MRI) scan results show three ring-enhancing lesions with surrounding edema in the right hemisphere. He is treated with dexamethasone, pyrimethamine, and sulfadiazine, with a resolution of his lesions and symptoms over 2 weeks. Serum toxoplasma titers are elevated.

Diagnosis

Central nervous system (CNS) toxoplasmosis associated with the acquired immune deficiency syndrome (AIDS).

The nervous system frequently is involved in HIV infection, and nervous system symptoms often dominate the clinical picture. HIV-related neurologic symptoms are caused by (a) direct infection of the nervous system, (b) secondary opportunistic infections of the nervous system, (c) tumors associated with AIDS, and (d) triggering of other processes such as inflammatory demyelinating peripheral neuropathies. Therapy of HIV and its complications also may result in neurologic abnormalities. No part of the nervous system is spared in patients with HIV infection. The goal of the physician is to suspect and identify HIV infection in patients who have particular nervous system conditions and to treat secondary infections accordingly. It is important to note that the use of highly active antiretroviral therapy (HAART) has markedly reduced the frequency of neurologic complications associated with HIV.

CENTRAL NERVOUS SYSTEM

HIV-Associated Dementia

Although many CNS manifestations of AIDS relate to secondary infections or tumors, the AIDS dementia complex is a specific clinical entity caused by direct brain infection with HIV. Note the following:

1. Many patients with AIDS eventually are afflicted with HIV-associated dementia (HAD). Most commonly, HAD develops after overt AIDS, although in many patients the dementia can present at the same time or before other manifestations of AIDS. In some patients, dementia may be the only clinical sign of HIV infection at the time of diagnosis. HAD remains one of the most common causes of dementia in patients younger than age 40 years. Therefore, HIV testing should be included in the evaluation of a young patient with unexplained dementia.

2. The incidence of HAD has declined from approximately 21% to almost 10% in the era of combination antiretroviral therapy.

3. The onset of dementia is usually insidious, although some patients may experience an abrupt, rapid worsening of their condition when the dementia appears suddenly over several days. In some patients, a rapidly accelerating dementia may occur in association with systemic illness.

4. Early symptoms and signs include cognitive changes (including forgetfulness, mental slowing, and poor concentration), motor difficulties (ataxia, leg weakness, deteriorating handwriting), behavioral abnormalities (apathy, social withdrawal, psychosis), and other findings such as headache and seizures. Cortical features such as aphasia, apraxia, alexia, and agraphia are less common. Mild disturbances of eye movements often are present.

5. The late manifestations include severe dementia, ataxia, motor weakness, incontinence, tremor, mutism, and frontal release signs (e.g., rooting reflex and grasp response).

6. Some patients have an associated retinopathy, myelopathy, or peripheral neuropathy.

7. *Laboratory studies.* HAD typically occurs in the setting of moderately severe immunosuppression. Mean CD4 counts are usually below 200 mm^3. Cerebrospinal fluid (CSF) is abnormal in approximately half of the patients and shows elevated protein levels, pleocytosis, and oligoclonal bands. Generally, HIV-1 ribonucleic acid levels in the CSF are elevated. Computed tomography (CT) or MRI scans are essential to rule out other focal conditions associated with AIDS (described later). Classic findings include atrophy, enlargement of cortical sulci, enlarged ventricles, and white-matter abnormalities. The detection of cerebral atrophy also has been reported among asymptomatic HIV patients and is therefore not diagnostic of HAD. The electroencephalogram results are usually normal in early stages of AIDS dementia complex.

8. Pathologic abnormalities result from direct viral invasion of the subcortical white matter, thalamus, and basal ganglia with relative sparing of the cerebral cortex. Neuron loss and astrocytosis are secondary effects of the viral invasion. An infiltration of macrophages is characteristic; these cells are believed to mediate much of the local damage via immunologic mechanisms. HAD is generally a diagnosis of exclusion. One must rule out other possible causes of dementia and delirium, including metabolic or drug-induced encephalopathy; cryptococcal meningitis; tuberculosis; intracranial mass lesion; neurosyphilis; and encephalitis secondary to herpes simplex virus (HSV), varicella zoster virus (VZV), and cytomegalovirus (CMV).

9. Most experts recommend initiation of combination antiretroviral therapy in patients with HAD. Data demonstrating consistent improvements in HAD following therapy, unfortunately, are limited.

Cerebral Toxoplasmosis

Cerebral toxoplasmosis is the most common cause of focal brain pathology (intracranial mass lesion) in patients with AIDS. It usually occurs when CD4+ counts are less than 100 cells/mm^3. It is particularly important to recognize it early because prompt initiation of therapy can ameliorate neurologic deficits. Note the following:

1. *Presenting clinical symptoms* and signs include focal manifestations, most commonly hemiparesis. In addition, patients may have seizures, aphasia, cranial nerve palsies, and ataxia. The most common nonfocal manifestations are confusion, lethargy, and headache. Patients occasionally have parkinsonism or choreoathetosis as a result of lesions in the basal ganglia,

2. The most sensitive *laboratory studies* include MRI or CT scan with contrast and blood serology. Ring-enhancing lesions are seen on both CT scan and MRI, although MRI imaging is more sensitive. Serum serologies almost always demonstrate elevated toxoplasma titers. Polymerase chain reaction (PCR) for toxoplasma in the CSF is sometimes helpful.

3. Most patients respond to *treatment* with pyrimethamine (200 mg initially followed by 25 to 75 mg po daily) and sulfadiazine (1 to 1.5 g every 6 hours) if treated early. Leucovorin (10 to 20 mg po daily) is necessary to prevent pyrimethamine-associated bone marrow suppression. Clindamycin is recommended in place of sulfadiazine when patients report sulfa allergies. Steroids should be used only in patients with significant mass effect and edema.

4. *Note:* Many patients with CNS toxoplasmosis may have underlying HAD. Thus, after resolution of the parasitic lesions, neurologic status may not return to normal. Simultaneous infections with other infectious agents are common.

5. Because cerebral toxoplasmosis is one of the more treatable neurologic complications of AIDS, a therapeutic trial for toxoplasmosis is indicated before brain biopsy in patients with suggestive radiographic findings and positive toxoplasma titers. Most patients demonstrate clinical and neuroradiographic improvement within 2 weeks of therapy. A failure to respond in 2 weeks warrants further diagnostic evaluation (including the possibility of stereotactic brain biopsy).

6. The other major cause of intracranial mass lesion in AIDS is primary CNS lymphoma. In many instances, it may not be possible to distinguish toxoplasmosis from lymphoma with-

out a brain biopsy. In general, CNS lymphomas are large, single lesions with variable rim enhancement. Lymphomas are encountered more commonly in the periventricular white matter and corpus callosum (see later in this chapter).

Other Central Nervous System Infections and Processes

Several other infections and pathologies can affect the brain in patients with HIV.

1. *Viral infections* include HSV, VZV, and CMV encephalitis; progressive multifocal leukoencephalopathy (PML; caused by the JC virus); and HIV or CMV retinitis. CMV retinitis can cause blindness rapidly and can be treated with systemic ganciclovir, valganciclovir, foscarnet, or cidofovir. Intraocular ganciclovir implants or injections also may stabilize the disease. Aggressive treatment of HIV with combination antiretroviral therapy is essential to prevent recurrence of CMV retinitis. An inflammatory vitritis may develop in patients with CMV retinitis who receive antiretroviral therapy as a result of immune reconstitution. The diagnosis of PML is supported by classic MRI findings (extensive nonenhancing white matter disease) and the detection of JC virus in the CSF by PCR.
2. *Nonviral infections* include tuberculosis, neurosyphilis, and fungal infections such as cryptococcus, *Candida,* and histoplasmosis.
3. *Neoplasms* also affect the brain in patients with AIDS: primary CNS lymphoma, systemic lymphoma with CNS involvement, and (rarely) Kaposi's sarcoma. Almost all primary CNS lymphomas are caused by Epstein-Barr virus in patients with advanced immunosuppression. CNS lymphoma is treated with radiation therapy and corticosteroids; many patients receive adjuvant chemotherapy. The prognosis of patients with CNS lymphoma traditionally has been poor, although prolonged survival in patients receiving combination antiretroviral therapy, radiation, and chemotherapy increasingly has been described.
4. *Stroke.* In some patients, *infarction or hemorrhage* may occur. Hemorrhage may be associated with CNS lymphoma, and infarction may be the consequence of arteritis, endocarditis, meningovascular syphilis, or tuberculous vasculopathy.

LEPTOMENINGES

1. The leptomeninges frequently are involved in AIDS. Examples include cryptococcal meningitis, aseptic meningitis, and lymphomatous meningitis. Diagnosis is based on lumbar puncture, CSF culture, and the detection of cryptococcal antigen in the serum and CSF.

2. Acute "aseptic" meningitis with headache, meningismus, cranial nerve palsies, and fever may occur at the time of seroconversion and probably represents primary infection with HIV. This process is generally self-limited. In some instances, a more indolent form of HIV-related meningitis occurs, presenting only as headache and low-grade pleocytosis. Acute HIV should remain in the differential diagnosis of all patients (especially those with appropriate risk factors) who present with unexplained aseptic meningitis.

SPINAL CORD

1. Spinal cord involvement in AIDS includes vacuolar myelopathy from HIV infection and viral myelitis caused by HSV, VZV, and CMV, among others. These viral syndromes present with spinal cord dysfunction (e.g., leg weakness and incontinence) and increased cells in the spinal fluid.

2. A specific syndrome may be seen with CMV infection of the cauda equina, with a rapid onset of painful paraplegia and bowel and bladder dysfunction. PCR testing of the CSF may yield an early diagnosis of CMV, leading to successful therapy.

3. *Myelopathy associated with human T-lymphotrophic virus type 1 (HTLV-1).* A separate syndrome associated with HTLV-1 affects the spinal cord. It is unrelated to HIV infection but is associated with another retrovirus, HTLV-1. This entity is termed tropical spastic paraparesis (TSP) or the HAM syndrome (HTLV-1-associated myelopathy). The HAM syndrome is endemic in southern Japan. Clinically, these patients have upper motor neuron spinal cord dysfunction associated with weakness, gait abnormalities, and spasticity. Patients also may have mild sensory and bladder disturbances. Diagnosis is based on elevated antibody titers to HTLV-1 virus in serum and spinal fluid. The cause of nervous system dysfunction is unclear. Treatment with steroids

may be of temporary benefit. Danazol, interferon, and plasmapheresis also have been used with mixed results.

PERIPHERAL NERVES

Peripheral nerve involvement may take the form of a sensory or sensorimotor polyneuropathy, inflammatory demyelinating polyneuropathy, mononeuropathy multiplex, and drug-related neuropathies.

1. *Sensory neuropathy* is seen in approximately 30% of patients. Symptoms include painful paresthesias affecting distal extremities. Symptoms occur late in the course of HIV infection. Treatment is symptomatic with drugs such as amitriptyline, nortriptyline, carbamazepine, gabapentin, or lamotrigine. Etiology is unclear and may relate to HIV infection of dorsal root ganglia plus nutritional and toxic factors.

2. *Inflammatory neuropathy* may be acute (Guillain-Barré syndrome) or chronic. In addition to increased CSF protein, these patients have significant CSF pleocytosis, which is generally not seen in typical cases of Guillain-Barré. Otherwise, this syndrome may mimic Guillain-Barré syndrome and may occur at HIV seroconversion. Patients respond to treatment with steroids or plasma exchange. Because plasma exchange is an accepted form of therapy for acute inflammatory polyneuropathy, all patients with this condition should be tested for HIV.

3. *Mononeuropathies* may be seen in HIV infection in association with the AIDS-related complex. Of patients with HIV infection, 5% to 10% will develop varicella zoster nerve root infection (radiculitis). The dermatomal rash is often diagnostic. Treatment with acyclovir, valacyclovir, or famciclovir is recommended. Postherpetic neuralgia is a possible complication.

4. *Drug-induced neuropathy.* Some drugs used to treat AIDS such as didanosine (ddI), stavudine (d4T), and zalcitabine (ddC) may cause a *dose-related peripheral neuropathy*. Discontinuation of the causative medication is essential for recovery. Antiretroviral-associated neuropathy is occasionally irreversible. An acute neuropathy associated with areflexia and ascending paresis has been associated with the development of lactic acidosis in patients treated with d4T and other antiretroviral medications. Mitochondrial damage is the postulated etiology for this condition (Table 25.1).

TABLE 25.1.   Neurologic Complications in Patients Infected with HIV-1[a]

BRAIN
Predominantly nonfocal
  HIV-associated dementia
  CMV encephalitis
  Metabolic encephalopathies
  HSV encephalitis
  Acute HIV-1-related encephalitis
Predominantly focal
  Cerebral toxoplasmosis
  Primary CNS lymphoma
  Progressive multifocal leukoencephalopathy
  Cryptococcoma
  Varicella zoster virus encephalitis
  Tuberculous brain abscess/tuberculoma
  Neurosyphilis (meningovascular)
  Vascular disorders
SPINAL CORD
Vacuolar myelopathy
Herpes zoster myelitis
HSV myelitis
MENINGES
Aseptic meningitis (HIV-1)
Cryptococcal meningitis
Metastatic lymphomatous meningitis
Tuberculous meningitis
Syphilitic meningitis
PERIPHERAL NERVE AND ROOT
Infectious
  Herpes zoster
  CMV polyradiculopathy
Virus or immune related
  Acute and chronic inflammatory demyelinating neuropathy
  Mononeuropathy
  Mononeuritis multiplex
  Autonomic neuropathy
  Sensorimotor polyneuropathy
  Distal painful sensory neuropathy
MUSCLE
Polymyositis and other myopathies

CMV, cytomegalovirus; CNS, central nervous system; HIV, human immunodeficiency virus; HSV, herpes simplex virus.
[a](Adapted from Brew BJ, Sidtis JJ, Petito CK, Price RW. The neurologic complications of AIDS and human immunodeficiency virus infection. In: Plum F, ed. *Advances in contemporary neurology*. Philadelphia: FA Davis, 1988, with permission.)

MUSCLE

Myositis has been described as a complication of HIV infection. Muscle biopsies have shown inflammatory changes including multinucleated giant cells plus HIV antigens in the muscle. Treatment with steroids may be helpful. Myopathy also may be related to the therapy of HIV, especially zidovudine (AZT). Discontinuation of AZT typically leads to rapid improvement.

Suggested Reading

Carpenter CCJ, Cooper DA, Fischl MA, et al. Antiretroviral therapy in adults: updated recommendations of the international AIDS Society—USA Panel. *JAMA* 2000;283:381–390.

Cohen B. Prognosis and response to therapy of cytomegalovirus encephalitis and meningomyelitis in AIDS. *Neurology* 1996;46: 444–450.

d'Arminio MA, Duca PG, Vago L et al. Decreasing incidence of CNS AIDS-defining events associated with antiretroviral therapy. *Neurology* 2000;54:1856–1859.

Dybul M, Fauci AS, Bartlett JG, et al. Guidelines for using antiretroviral agents among HIV-infected adults and adolescents. *Ann Intern Med* 2002;137:381–433.

Enting RH, Hoetelmans RM, Lange JM, et al. Antiretroviral drugs and the central nervous system. *AIDS* 1998;12:1941–1955.

Flinn IW, Ambinder RF. AIDS primary central nervous system lymphoma. *Curr Opin Oncol* 1996;8:373–376.

Holland NR, Power C, Mathews VP, et al. Cytomegalovirus encephalitis in acquired immunodeficiency syndrome (AIDS). *Neurology* 1994;44: 507–514.

Hollander H, McGuire D, Burack JH. Diagnostic lumbar puncture in HIV-infected patients: analysis of 138 cases. *Am J Med* 1994;96: 223–228.

Holloway RG, Mushlin AI. Intracranial mass lesions in acquired immunodeficiency syndrome: using decision analysis to determine the effectiveness of stereotactic brain biopsy. *Neurology* 1996;46: 1010–1015.

Lange DJ. AAEM Minimonograph #41: Neuromuscular disease associated with HIV-1 infection. *Muscle Nerve* 1994;17:16.

Masur H, Kaplan JE, Holmes KK, et al. Recommendations of the U.S. Public Health Service and the Infectious Diseases Society of America. *Ann Intern Med* 2002;137:435–478.

Palella FJ, Delaney KM, Moorman AC, et al. HIV Outpatient Study Investigators. Declining morbidity and mortality among patients with advanced human immunodeficiency virus infection. *N Engl J Med* 1998;338:853.

Price RW. Neurological complications of HIV infection. *Lancet* 1996;348: 445–452.

Sacktor N, Lyles RH, Skolasky R, et al. HIV-associated neurologic disease incidence changes: Multicenter AIDS Cohort Study, 1990–1998. *Neurology* 2001; 56:257–260.

Treisman GJ, Kaplin AI. Neurologic and psychiatric complications of antiretroviral agents. *AIDS* 2002;16:1201–1215.

Van der horst CM, Saag MS, Cloud GA, et al. Treatment of cryptococcal meningitis associated with the acquired immunodeficiency syndrome. *N Engl J Med* 1997;337:15–21.

Chapter 26

Neurology of Uremia

Case

A 64-year-old man with end-stage renal failure undergoing hemodialysis develops a generalized headache that is worse after each dialysis treatment. He often is confused for a few hours after each treatment. One day as he is coming in for dialysis treatment, he is noted to be unable to walk and incontinent of urine. A computed tomography (CT) scan leads to a surgical procedure after which his mental status returns to normal.

Diagnosis

Bilateral, chronic subdural hematomas associated with uremia and dialysis.

MENTAL STATUS CHANGES

One of the most common features of renal failure is an altered mental status. It may range from irritability and difficulty in concentration (e.g., performing "serial 7s") to actual psychotic reactions. Mental status changes in uremia fluctuate; periods of confusion are interspersed with periods of lucidity. *Acute changes in mental status* generally are encountered after dialysis when there have been rapid electrolyte shifts, although actual electrolyte values are improved ("dysequilibrium syndrome"). Metabolic shifts in brain pH or urea often lag behind the changes in the blood values. Slowly developing renal failure causes fewer cognitive changes than does rapidly developing failure. Acute uremia may be accompanied by tremor, fasciculations, myoclonus, chorea, or convulsions. Patients undergoing dialysis are at risk for complex partial status epilepticus, and patients with an unexplained encephalopathy should have an electroencephalogram (EEG).

EEG changes are usual with an altered mental status, and slowing usually parallels the degree of metabolic encephalopathy. Most patients with a blood urea nitrogen level higher than 60 mg/100 mL have EEG abnormalities (generalized slowing). With complex partial status, continuous focal seizure activity or rhythmic slowing may be seen.

Although most mental status changes in uremia are not secondary to treatable nervous system disease, keep other possibilities in mind:

1. *Infection.* Listeria, fungal, or other central nervous system (CNS) pathogens are not uncommon in patients with uremia. When there is unexplained confusion or fever in the patient with uremia, after performing a CT scan or magnetic resonance imaging (MRI) to rule out subdural hematoma or other mass lesion, perform a lumbar puncture (LP). Remember to do an India ink preparation for *Cryptococcus* or test for cryptococcal antigen if there are cells in the cerebrospinal fluid (CSF) (see Chapter 30).

2. *Subdural hematoma.* Patients with uremia have an increased bleeding tendency, and subdural collections may develop with mild head trauma or during dialysis. If a subdural hematoma is suspected because of lateralizing signs or persistent lethargy with headache, obtain a CT or MRI scan.

3. *Hypertensive encephalopathy.* Hypertension frequently accompanies uremia, and hypertensive crisis may mimic the clinical features of uremic encephalopathy. Look for markedly elevated blood pressure, papilledema, and retinal hemorrhages. MRI changes that are bilateral, subcortical, and suggestive of edema may be dramatic and are reversible with resolution of the hypertensive encephalopathy. Patients with cyclosporine toxicity may be especially sensitive to mild hypertension, which can cause a reversible posterior hemisphere leukoencephalopathy. Clinically, these patients present with confusion, lethargy, and visual symptoms. They respond to lowering blood pressure and withholding cyclosporine.

SEIZURES

Seizures are a common feature of renal disease. They signify different processes, depending on the type (generalized or focal) and the clinical setting (e.g., postdialysis). Patients with *acute anuria* may develop tonic-clonic seizures on the 8th to 11th day of renal failure or with the onset of diuresis and subsequent rapid electrolyte shifts.

Tonic-clonic seizures also appear late in the course of *chronic renal disease* and frequently are associated with abnormal blood chemistries: acidosis, hypokalemia, and hyponatremia. No one abnormal electrolyte is associated consistently with seizures, but the greater the potassium/calcium ratio, the greater the risk of seizure.

Seizures are common *after dialysis* because of fluid and electrolyte shifts. Seizures may occur as a result of hypertensive encephalopathy, which is common in untreated uremia.

Remember, generalized tonic-clonic seizures caused by metabolic disorders may not respond to antiepileptic drugs; consider dialysis and aggressive management of the metabolic abnormalities. This is especially important when status epilepticus is present.

Treatment of Tonic-Clonic Seizures

1. The drug of choice is *phenytoin,* which is metabolized by the liver—not kidney—and is not removed during dialysis. Administer 15 to 18 mg/kg intravenously over 30 to 45 minutes if immediate therapeutic levels are needed, then 300 to 400 mg daily. Follow the phenytoin levels, including the free (unbound) phenytoin level, which is increased in renal failure. Fos-phenytoin also may be used.
2. *Generalized or multifocal* seizures (one side, then the other) occurring during metabolic flux (dialysis, diuresis) are generally self-limited. Treat with phenytoin. When the patient's condition has stabilized, anticonvulsants may be withdrawn.
3. Patients with persistent *focal* seizures should be worked up for subdural hematoma, tumor, infection, or infarction with CT scan or MRI, LP, and EEG. Patients may have tiny areas of cortical hemorrhage that account for focal seizures.
4. Check for predisposing electrolyte disturbances, and correct where appropriate.

PERIPHERAL NEUROPATHY

Early

Patients often develop a "restless leg syndrome" as an early sign of uremic neuropathy. The legs feel uncomfortable when the patient is still, and relief occurs after ambulation. Another early neuropathic syndrome consists of painful, burning paresthesias of the feet similar to those seen in alcoholics and associated with dietary insufficiency. Resolution may follow proper diet and vitamin supplements.

Late

A more severe peripheral neuropathy develops over weeks to months and is not diet-dependent. Check for distal loss of all sensory modalities (pinprick, position, vibration). The legs are affected significantly more than the arms. The neuropathy is motor and sensory and may lead to actual paraplegia (at this stage the arms also may become involved). Treatment is difficult. Although dialysis helps somewhat, it is generally ineffective; renal transplantation reverses the neuropathy. Nerve conduction studies are abnormal in most patients with renal disease, regardless of whether they have symptomatic neuropathy.

OTHER NEUROLOGIC FEATURES OF UREMIA

Dialysis may precipitate convulsions or a toxic encephalopathy. In this "reverse urea syndrome," urea leaves the brain more slowly than it leaves the blood; fluid, thus, is drawn into the brain, resulting in acute swelling. The encephalopathy usually clears in 24 to 48 hours. Remember, subdural hematoma sometimes follows dialysis.

Asterixis frequently accompanies uremic encephalopathy, as do muscle fasciculations and myoclonus. *Muscle cramps* may occur and generally are unrelated to a specific electrolyte abnormality, although they are more frequent when water intoxication is present. Chvostek's sign may be positive in uremia; it is correlated with the acidosis and elevated potassium/calcium ratio rather than with decreased calcium alone. There may be mild proximal muscle weakness (Table 26.1).

TABLE 26.1.   Signs and Symptoms of Uremic Encephalopathy[a]

Early	Moderate	Severe
Anorexia	Vomiting	Itching
Nausea	Sluggishness	Disorientation
Insomnia	Easy fatigue	Confusion
Restlessness	Drowsiness	Bizarre behavior
Decreased attention span	Sleep inversion	Slurring of speech
Inability to manage ideas	Volatile emotions	Hypothermia
Decreased sexual interest	Paranoia	Myoclonus
	Decreased cognitive function	Asterixis convulsions
		Stupor coma
	Inability to decipher abstractions	
	Decreased sexual performance	

[a](From Fraser CL, Arieff AI. Nervous system complications of uremia. *Ann Intern Med* 1988;109:143–153, with permission.)

Uremic amaurosis has been reported with the acute development of blindness; this may be related to focal cerebral edema. Complete recovery usually occurs. A reversible posterior leukoencephalopathy that may be the cause of this syndrome has been described.

Cerebral emboli may occur during the declotting of shunts used for hemodialysis. *Dialysis dementia* has been reported in patients with uremia; it represents a subacutely progressive neurologic deterioration in patients undergoing hemodialysis. It consists of dementia, myoclonus, speech disorders, neuropsychiatric abnormalities, gait abnormalities, and EEG changes (periodic sharp waves or spike and wave). Aluminum intoxication appears to be an important factor. Clinical and EEG improvement may follow treatment with diazepam or other anticonvulsants. This disorder has become rarer with removal of aluminum from most dialysate solutions.

Cranial nerve abnormalities in uremia may cause nystagmus, facial weakness, dizziness, and hearing loss. Symptoms caused by the uremia must be differentiated from those caused by ototoxic/nephrotoxic drugs.

Carpal tunnel syndrome is common in patients undergoing hemodialysis. Focal neuropathies sometimes are associated with vascular graft placement, occurring distal to the graft site, and are related to vascular steal phenomena as a result of the graft.

Transplant patients being treated with *cyclosporine* may experience tremors and paresthesias early after transplantation, related to high-dose cyclosporine, which usually resolves when the cyclosporine dose is decreased.

Some patients treated for *transplant rejection with OKT3* monoclonal antibody may experience an aseptic meningitis syndrome (headaches, stiff neck) with pleocytosis in the CSF, related to the monoclonal antibody. Rarely, a stupor or coma may occur. A small percentage of patients suffer nerve injuries during the transplantation procedure. CNS infections, particularly fungal or viral infections, have been reported in renal transplant patients.

Uremic myopathy may occur. This often is associated with bone pain and tenderness and is similar to that found in primary hyperparathyroidism and osteomalacia.

Suggested Reading

Bruno A, Adams HP. Neurologic problems in renal transplant recipients. *Neurol Clin* 1989;7:617–627.

Burn DJ, Bates D. Neurology and the kidney. *J Neurol Neurosurg Psychiatry* 1998;65(6):810–821.

De Deyn PP, Saxena VK, Abts H, et al. Clinical and pathophysiological aspects of neurological complications in renal failure. *Acta Neurol Belgica* 1992;92:191–206.

Fraser CL, Arieff AI. Nervous system complications in uremia. *Ann Intern Med* 1988;109:143–153.

Lockwood AH. Neurologic complications of renal disease. *Neurol Clin* 1989;7:617–627.

Smogorzewski MJ. Central nervous dysfunction in uremia. *Am J Kidney Dis* 2001;38(4 Suppl 1):S122–S128.

Chapter 27

Neurology of Alcoholism

Case

The chief executive officer of a small company is admitted for an appendectomy. Two days postsurgery, he experiences two generalized tonic-clonic seizures that occur within 15 minutes of each other. The patient is jittery, anxious, and sweating, with a moderate tachycardia. He admits that he drinks three large Manhattans every night and more on weekends. Results of an electroencephalogram (EEG) and magnetic resonance imaging scan with gadolinium are normal.

Diagnosis

Alcohol withdrawal seizures.

SEIZURES

Seizures are common in the person who is an alcoholic and represent at least two different phenomena. It is important to distinguish the two types of "alcoholic seizures" because treatment and workup are different.

Alcoholic Withdrawal Seizures

Alcoholic withdrawal seizures are brief, self-limited, generalized seizures secondary to abstinence from alcohol or a reduction in the usual intake. They do not represent a true convulsive disorder and most occur 12 to 48 hours after cessation of drinking (rarely after 96 hours). A night's sleep without alcohol may be enough to precipitate a seizure. Remember, alcohol withdrawal seizures can occur in the "businessman drinker" who comes to the hospital for other reasons, often for an operation. Alcohol withdrawal seizures tend to appear in groups of two or three and then stop. The patient is usually tremulous and jittery. The interictal EEG in these patients is usually normal, and if the history is characteristic, the patient requires no further neurologic workup or anticonvulsant medication. Often a patient is placed on anticonvulsant medications in the hospital after the first seizure, but when it becomes apparent that it was a "withdrawal seizure," anticonvulsants are tapered and discontinued. Patients with alcoholic withdrawal seizures are markedly sensitive to photic stimulation during EEG. They are also at a higher risk for developing delirium tremens (DTs).

Seizures Precipitated by Alcohol

These alcohol-*induced* seizures are usually focal and reflect an intrinsic central nervous system (CNS) lesion. Seizures of this type may occur during the period of intoxication. Such patients generally have an abnormal EEG; they require a basic neurologic workup for seizure and treatment with anticonvulsants. Focal seizures in the alcoholic often represent posttraumatic epilepsy caused by multiple falls. Remember that focal seizures represent CNS pathology, and alcoholics are especially prone to subdural hematoma and meningitis. Persistently focal seizures in an alcoholic should be considered to be caused by a subdural hematoma until proved otherwise. Of course, an alcoholic has the same risk for a brain tumor or atrioventricular malformation as does the general population.

Remember, the questions to answer when treating the seizure of an alcoholic: Was the seizure focal or generalized? When did it occur in relation to drinking?

ALCOHOLIC TREMULOUSNESS—DELIRIUM TREMENS

The spectrum of alcohol withdrawal symptoms ranges from mild tremulousness to fatal DTs. The underlying physiology in these states is related to abstinence from alcohol, not to specific dietary or vitamin insufficiency. Similar withdrawal states can occur after stopping other CNS depressants (e.g., barbiturates, diazepam). DTs and withdrawal seizures can be produced in normal people with good diets who are placed on large amounts of alcohol and then withdrawn. Seizures are a point on the spectrum of withdrawal symptomatology. An alcoholic who stops drinking is subject to the following:

1. *Tremulousness* is one of the first signs of alcohol withdrawal, beginning approximately 8 hours after cessation of drinking (often after a night's sleep) and reaching its peak at 24 hours. The patient is jittery, startles easily, and often shows a gross irregular tremor of the hands. There are signs of sympathetic overactivity, with increased sweating and heart rate. Although these symptoms are most severe at 24 hours, it may take 7 to 10 days before the patient is back to normal. Drinkers who suffer from tremulousness when waking in the morning may take a drink to "calm their nerves."

2. *Seizures* (discussed earlier).

3. *Hallucinations* appear during the withdrawal period and are commonly visual, although they may be auditory. Sometimes the patient hallucinates in the presence of an otherwise clear sensorium.

4. *DTs* complete the spectrum. This serious reaction occurs approximately 72 to 96 hours after cessation of drinking. Those who have had a chronic period of drinking before cessation experience the most severe form of DTs. Patients suffer from tremulousness, hallucinations, and marked autonomic hyperactivity (tachycardia, hyperhidrosis, fever, dilated pupils). DTs are a relatively uncommon sequelae of alcoholic withdrawal but can be fatal; they often are preceded by an alcoholic withdrawal seizure. The mortality rate is significant if DTs are untreated because of cardiovascular collapse, self-injury, electrolyte disorders, and infections.

Treatment of Delirium Tremens

Treatment consists primarily of supportive care. Adequate diet and vitamins have no effect on the course of alcohol withdrawal but must be given to prevent other complications. Pay careful attention to fluid and electrolyte balance (several liters of saline a day may be needed), correct hypoglycemia, and search thoroughly for underlying disease (e.g., subdural hematoma, pneumonia, or meningitis). These diseases are not uncommon and often are the factors that make DTs fatal. Treat with diazepam, 10 mg intravenously (IV), then 5 mg or more every 5 minutes up to 40 mg IV until the patient is calm, with maintenance of 5 mg or more IV or intramuscularly (IM) every 1 to 4 hours as needed. Other benzodiazepines, such as lorazepam and chlordiazepoxide, also may be used. There is no evidence that steroids are of benefit. Atenolol, a β-adrenergic blocker, is sometimes helpful in selected patients with the alcohol withdrawal syndrome. It may be impossible to prevent DTs, but one can decrease the severity of agitation with medication; by controlling fluid and electrolyte balance, the chances for recovery are good.

VITAMIN DEFICIENCY SYNDROMES AND ALCOHOLISM

In addition to the alcohol withdrawal syndrome, there is a group of vitamin deficiency syndromes seen almost exclusively in alcoholics. These also appear in nonalcoholics with poor diets or with cachexia associated with cancer.

Wernicke's Encephalopathy

Wernicke's encephalopathy is an important deficiency disorder caused by a lack of thiamine, which is associated with changes in the thalamus and brainstem. It causes a classic triad:

1. *Oculomotor changes.* Look for nystagmus on horizontal or vertical gaze, sixth nerve palsies that are generally bilateral, and paralysis of conjugate gaze. In severe forms there may be total ophthalmoplegia.
2. *Gait difficulties.* Check for ataxia: a wide-based gait, falling, or inability to walk or stand. Limb ataxia (finger-to-arm testing) is usually absent.
3. *Mental symptoms.* Patients usually manifest a quiet, apathetic, confused state. *Korsakoff's psychosis* is an extension of the mental symptoms of Wernicke's disease and becomes apparent later if the Wernicke's syndrome is untreated. The main feature is a marked disorder of memory with confabulation. The patient is unable to learn new material such as the doctor's name or who visited 10 minutes earlier; the patient often confabulates or "fills in" with false information. CT scans in chronic alcoholics often show evidence of cerebral and cerebellar atrophy.

Remember, Wernicke's encephalopathy often is underdiagnosed and may not present with all parts of the classic triad. Consider Wernicke's encephalopathy in confused patients who have nutritional deficiencies of any type. Treat early and aggressively. In addition to the previously mentioned triad, thiamine deficiency can produce dysautonomia, including cardiac failure, and electrocardiography abnormalities.

Treatment consists of thiamine (50 mg IV and 50 mg IM) to improve the oculomotor dysfunction and to prevent the development of Korsakoff's psychosis. Gastrointestinal malabsorption in alcoholics makes oral treatment unreliable. The 50-mg IM dose should be repeated daily until the patient resumes a normal diet. Occasionally, larger doses may be needed, initially to improve oculomotor dysfunction. Be careful when giving intravenous fluids to alcoholics; glucose may cause depletion of thiamine stores and precipitate Wernicke's syndrome. Thus, add thiamine to the intravenous solutions.

Wernicke's syndrome also can occur in nonalcoholics who depend on parenteral alimentation (e.g., surgical or burn unit patients) or in patients with malnutrition as a result of starvation, renal failure, cancer, or acquired immune deficiency syndrome.

Polyneuropathy

Polyneuropathy occurs in alcoholics secondary to nutritional factors and also may be related in part to the toxic effects of alcohol. Most patients are asymptomatic but lose ankle and sometimes knee jerks. When symptoms occur, they consist of burning, painful feet, with mild distal weakness. The feet may be so sensitive that even the touch of the bed covers is painful. In severe cases, the weakness may progress to wrist-drop and foot-drop. Polyneuropathy and Wernicke's syndrome often occur in the same patient.

Treatment consists of improving the diet, completely abstaining from alcohol, and adding vitamin supplements. Some clinicians give phenytoin or carbamazepine during the acute stage. Recovery is slow but usually occurs with abstinence from alcohol and proper diet.

OTHER NEUROLOGIC COMPLICATIONS OF ALCOHOLISM

Cerebellar degeneration affects men more frequently than women and midline structures more than the cerebellar hemispheres.

Thus, there is a wide-based gait with truncal instability and less prominent limb ataxia. The symptoms appear over weeks to months, although they may come on acutely. The acutely occurring syndrome has a better prognosis and may not represent actual cerebellar structural damage, as does the chronic form. Treatment consists of dietary and vitamin support. Abstinence from alcohol is crucial.

Some patients may have slowly developing *myopathy* with proximal muscle weakness, often in conjunction with alcoholic cardiac myopathy. There is an acute form with muscle pain, weakness, and elevated creatinine phosphokinase and myoglobinuria. Treatment is symptomatic. Rare complications of alcoholism or malnutrition include *central pontine myelinolysis* and the *Marchiafava-Bignami corpus callosum syndrome* .

Chronic alcoholic hallucinosis may occur after many bouts of acute alcoholic hallucinosis and may be confused with schizophrenia.

Note: Alcohol *intoxication* consists of varying degrees of excitement, disinhibition, slurred speech, unsteady gait, and drowsiness leading to stupor or coma. Idiosyncratic excitement may occur in some individuals with aggressive and assaultive behavior. Alcoholic "blackouts" refer to episodes in which time is lost during alcohol intoxication. Treatment of stupor or coma caused by alcohol ingestion is primarily supportive, although hemodialysis may be considered for high blood alcohol concentrations.

Neurologic Complications of Other Drugs

The neurologic complications of drugs other than alcohol are beyond the scope of this text. A few points about other drugs are as follows:

1. Opioids cause euphoria, sedation, nausea, sweating, constipation, and analgesia. They also cause miosis, which is a useful sign. Overdose causes coma, respiratory depression, and pinpoint but reactive pupils.
2. Stimulant medications such as amphetamines and cocaine cause increased motor activity and physical endurance. Overdose may cause hypertension, tachycardia, headache, chest pain, and fever. Delirium, cardiac arrhythmias, seizures, and strokes may occur.
3. Sedative agents such as barbiturates and benzodiazepines cause sedation and respiratory suppression. Withdrawal of

such agents may cause seizures, tremors, and agitation, all of which may be suppressed by the institution of barbiturate or benzodiazepines.

4. Marijuana causes a euphoric state, disinhibition, and postural hypotension. Fatal overdose has not been reported.

5. Hallucinogens such as lysergic acid diethylamide cause perceptual distortions, hallucinosis, and sense of depersonalization; some patients experience "flashbacks, " vivid recurrence of drug symptoms long after the cessation of drug use.

6. Glue sniffing and use of other inhalants such as lighter fluid cause symptoms such as euphoria, somnolence, hallucinations, and seizures.

7. Phencyclidine (PCP) causes stimulant symptoms, in addition to paranoia, hallucinosis, rhabdomyolysis, and seizures. Symptoms can persist for hours to days.

Suggested Reading

Breiter HC, Gollub RI, Weisskoff RM, et al. Acute effects of cocaine on human brain activity and emotion. *Neuron* 1997;19:591–611.

Brust JCM. *Neurologic aspects of substance abuse.* Boston: Butterworth-Heinmann, 1993.

Freilich RJ, Byrne E. Alcohol and drug abuse. *Curr Opin Neurol Neurosurg* 1992;5:391–395.

O'Connor PG, Schottenfeld RS. Patients with alcohol problems. *N Engl J Med* 1998;338(9):592–602

Reuter JB. Wernicke's encephalopathy. *N Engl J Med* 1985;312:1035–1038.

Saitz R, Mayo-Smith MF, Roberts MS. Individualized treatment for alcohol withdrawal: a randomized double-blind controlled trial. *JAMA* 1994;272:519–523.

Wrenn KD, Slovis CM. Neurologic complications of alcoholism. *Emerg Med Clin North Am* 1990;8:835–858.

Chapter 28

Neurology of Other Systemic Diseases

Case

A 57-year-old woman complains of weakness when getting out of a chair and a hoarse voice. She has been losing hair and gaining weight, and friends tell her she is "slowing down." On examination, her reflexes are hypoactive, and her muscles feel doughy to the touch.

Diagnosis

Hypothyroidism with myopathy and neuropathy.

Many systemic diseases exhibit neurologic manifestations, as described in preceding chapters regarding the neurology of diabetes, malignancy, uremia, and alcohol, as well as in the stroke chapter. The physician must recognize the many neurologic complications that accompany systemic disorders and treat them accordingly.

CARDIAC DISEASE

Cardiac abnormalities can cause reduced cerebral perfusion or emboli that lead to neurologic sequelae. The severity of neurologic manifestations of reduced cardiac output varies with the rate and extent of decreased cerebral perfusion. Ischemic brain injury can lead to seizures, cerebral edema, loss of consciousness, amnesia, and dementia.

Emboli from the heart are the cause of 15% of ischemic strokes. Thrombi, from which emboli emerge, may develop from a left atrial or ventricular mural thrombus, an intracardiac tumor, bacterial and nonbacterial endocarditis, or the systemic and right heart circulation via intracardiac shunts (paradoxic emboli). Conditions that predispose the patient to develop such emboli include atrial fibrillation, acute and chronic ischemic heart disease, and valvular heart diseases (rheumatic and prosthetic). Mitral annulus calcification, calcific aortic stenosis, and atrial septal aneurysm also can cause cerebral emboli.

Hemorrhagic strokes may occur after an occluding embolus and may result from reperfusion of tissue infarcted by the embolus. Young patients without evidence of cerebrovascular disease should be suspected of having a cardiac cause of stroke. Electrocardiogram (ECG), echocardiography, prolonged ECG monitoring to identify arrhythmias, and transesophageal echocardiography are helpful tests for detecting the cause of cardiogenic stroke. Transthoracic echocardiography has a low yield in showing cardiac sources of embolism because most of the structures in embolus formation are in the posterior areas of the heart (i.e., atria)

Anticoagulation therapy reduces the risk of embolism in atrial fibrillation, rheumatic mitral stenosis, and cardiomyopathy with ventricular thrombi. After a myocardial infarction (MI), patients are at risk for stroke, especially with anterior wall infarction. If echocardiography detects a developing thrombus, anticoagulation reduces the risk of post-MI stroke by at least 60%.

Anoxic encephalopathy, which is lack of oxygen to the brain, often occurs in the setting of cardiac arrest. Mild degrees of hypoxemia cause inattention, drowsiness, and impaired judgment, and in patients with prior deficits, hypoxemia may make symptoms worse. Anoxic injury may cause a variety of symptoms that can occur individually or in combination and include the following: (a) cortical damage or a watershed infarction leading to dementia or visual agnosia, (b) cerebellar injury causing ataxia, (c) memory impairment caused by injury to the mesial thalamus and hippocampus, and (d) choreoathetosis or a parkinsonian syndrome. Coma, stupor, or persistent vegetative state may occur with severe diffuse injury. No specific treatment, other than resumption of oxygenation, has been found helpful. Occasionally, patients with watershed infarctions have the "man in the barrel" syndrome, with weakness of shoulder girdle muscles sparing the hands, so the affected person cannot abduct the arms. This pattern results from infarction affecting the shoulder region in the cortex, which lies between anterior and middle cerebral territories in the watershed zone.

ENDOCRINE DISEASE

1. *Thyroid disease. Hyperthyroid* patients often complain of nervousness, fatigue, and irritability. They may have seizures, tremor, and chorea and usually have brisk tendon reflexes. They also may develop ophthalmopathy including proptosis and ophthalmoplegia; myopathy with proximal muscle weakness and wasting is common. Encephalopathy may occur with Hashimoto's thyroiditis. Patients have confusion, altered consciousness, and seizures associated with increased antithyroid antibodies and may respond to steroid therapy. *Hypothyroid* patients complain of fatigue and exhibit apathy, decreased attention, and slowness in answering questions. Myxedema coma is rare and carries a high mortality rate. Some patients may develop seizures, obstructive sleep apnea, ataxia, or sensorineural hearing loss. Myopathy is common, including exertional pain, stiffness, and cramps. Creatine phosphokinase (CPK) usually is elevated. On physical examination, hypoactive reflexes with a delayed relaxation time usually can be demonstrated. Reflexes may be pendular (i.e., the leg swings to and fro more often than normal if allowed to swing freely). Check for hyperthyroidism in patients with action tremor; check for hypothyroidism in patients with carpal tunnel syndrome.

2. *Parathyroid.* Patients with *hyperparathyroidism* often display psychiatric symptoms such as those associated with mania, schizophrenia, or depression. Myopathy is common. Patients with *hypoparathyroidism* may have psychiatric symptoms similar to those seen in hyperparathyroidism, and seizures can occur from hypocalcemia, particularly in hyperparathyroid patients after adenoma removal. Hypocalcemia and hypomagnesemia can cause tetany. To elicit latent tetany, have the patient hyperventilate and tap the facial nerve, causing facial muscle contraction (Chvostek's sign), or occlude venous return from an arm, resulting in carpopedal spasm

(Trousseau's sign). Laryngeal spasm also may occur in this setting.

3. *Glucocorticoids.* Myopathy is common with corticosteroid therapy, and myalgia may accompany the weakness. Treatment involves tapering or use of alternate-day steroids, alternate forms of immunosuppression, or nonfluorinated steroids. Patients with Cushing's syndrome may experience psychiatric symptoms. Patients with Addison's disease and patients after withdrawal from steroids may experience acute confusional states or psychosis. Seizures can occur from hyponatremia.

FLUID AND ELECTROLYTE DISTURBANCES

1. *Sodium.* Manifestations of *hyponatremia* range from confusion to coma. Patients also may experience convulsions, hemiparesis, ataxia, tremor, aphasia, and corticospinal tract signs. Sodium must be corrected to 120 to 125 mEq/L when convulsions are present because such patients have a high mortality if this is not done. However, too rapid correction of hyponatremia may result in central pontine myelinolysis. Patients with subarachnoid hemorrhage and hyponatremia should not be fluid restricted because their hyponatremia, previously attributed to the syndrome of inappropriate antidiuretic hormone secretion, actually is associated with volume depletion. *Hypernatremia* causes symptoms from lethargy to coma, seizures, rigidity, tremor, myoclonus, asterixis, and chorea. It may be seen in association with fluid loss and in the elderly from dehydration. Hyperosmolar states may be associated with cerebral edema.

2. *Potassium.* *Hypokalemia* causes muscle weakness, myalgia, and fatigability. With very low potassium levels (less than 2.5 mEq/L), rhabdomyolysis and myoglobinuria may occur. Rapid recovery occurs with potassium replacement. Occasionally, this state is mistaken for Guillain-Barré syndrome. *Hyperkalemia* is cardiotoxic and rarely is associated with neurologic symptoms before the heart is affected.

3. *Calcium.* *Hypercalcemia* may occur in patients with malignant neoplasms (particularly breast and lung cancer and multiple myeloma) and in patients with hyperparathyroidism. Patients may experience lethargy, muscle weakness, fatiga-

bility, confusion, headache, convulsions, and coma. Patients with hyperparathyroidism often display psychiatric symptoms (see Parathyroid). *Hypocalcemia* is less common but is seen in patients with renal failure. Acute hypocalcemia most often occurs after thyroid or parathyroid surgery and is a complication of acute pancreatitis. Patients are agitated and may experience delirium, hallucinations, and psychosis. Seizures may occur. Hypocalcemia (or hypomagnesemia) can cause tetany.

4. *Magnesium.* With decreased magnesium, patients are irritable and confused and may experience tetany, convulsions, tremor, and myoclonus. They are hyperreflexic and demonstrate a Chvostek sign. Treatment of convulsions is with parental magnesium. *Hypermagnesemia* is rare and occurs with increased intake in the setting of decreased renal function. It causes lethargy and confusion, and muscle paralysis may result.

GASTROINTESTINAL DISEASE

1. *Hepatic encephalopathy.* Mental changes range from delirium to coma. Tremor, paratonia, asterixis, and hyperactive reflexes also are seen. Asterixis is a sudden cessation of muscle activity and is best seen by having the patient hold the hands extended at the wrists with the arms outstretched. The hands suddenly fall forward, then rise up again. It also may be seen in other metabolic disorders or with drug intoxications. The electroencephalogram demonstrates slowing and triphasic waves. Serum ammonia levels may be increased but do not correlate well with the presence of hepatic encephalopathy. Causes of encephalopathy include toxins and metabolic derangements. Gastrointestinal (GI) bleeding frequently precipitates a bout of hepatic encephalopathy. If focal neurologic symptoms occur in the setting of hepatic encephalopathy, look for a structural lesion. Hepatic encephalopathy may unmask previously asymptomatic lesions such as a chronic subdural hematoma. Imaging also may demonstrate subarachnoid or intracerebral hemorrhage, related to coagulopathy associated with hepatic disease.

2. *Malabsorption.* Several GI disorders are associated with malabsorption (e.g., inflammatory bowel disease, postgastric

resection). This may lead to thiamine deficiency and Wernicke's encephalopathy or Korsakoff's psychosis (see Chapter 27). Cyanocobalamin (vitamin B_{12}) can be deficient in a vegetarian's diet, after gastric resection, with intrinsic factor deficiency (pernicious anemia), in a patient without a functional terminal ileum, or with pancreatic insufficiency. Patients experience paresthesias, sensory loss, ataxia, and dementia. Patients who lack vitamin B_6 can develop peripheral neuropathy. Those with vitamin A deficiency have an increased risk of night blindness; inadequate amounts of vitamin E cause neuropathy and cerebellar dysfunction.

3. *Wilson's disease. Wilson's disease* is an autosomal recessive disorder of copper metabolism manifested by cirrhosis and degeneration of the caudate and putamen. Patients may have tremor, dysarthria, dementia, and psychiatric symptoms. Patients have a Kayser-Fleischer ring on ophthalmologic examination, decreased serum ceruloplasmin level, and increased copper concentration on liver biopsy.

4. *Other disorders. Chronic hepatocerebral degeneration* is a slowly progressive neurologic syndrome manifested by chronic intermittent episodes of hepatic encephalopathy seen in patients with hepatic disease. Permanent neurologic signs and symptoms may result, including tremor, ataxia, dysarthria, nystagmus, dementia, choreoathetosis, pyramidal tract signs, and grasp reflexes. Patients with portal-systemic shunts may experience a myelopathy associated with dysarthria. The etiology is unclear.

Note: Inflammatory bowel disease may be associated with several neurologic problems including peripheral neuropathies, myelopathy, myopathy, myasthenia, and cerebrovascular disorders. *Whipple's disease* may cause an encephalopathy and occasionally a movement disorder called oculomyorhythmia, with oscillatory eye and mouth movements.

HEMATOLOGIC DISEASE

1. *Anemia.* Common symptoms of anemia include fatigue, headache, and lightheadedness. Individuals with sickle cell anemia may develop stroke, convulsions, or a change in level of consciousness. Patients with chronic hematologic diseases characterized by bone marrow failure or hemolytic anemia

have extramedullary hematopoiesis that may involve meninges surrounding the spinal cord and brain, leading to myelopathy or intracranial mass lesions.

2. *Hyperviscosity.* Patients with hyperviscosity may experience headache, lightheadedness, tinnitus, stupor, convulsions, or stroke. Causative diseases include polycythemia vera, leukocytosis, and paraproteinemias with Waldenstrom's macroglobulinemia and multiple myeloma. Patients with leukemia have a high incidence of intracerebral hemorrhage, and patients with paraproteinemia have reduced cerebral blood flow, peripheral neuropathies, mononeuritis multiplex, and cerebral infarction.

3. *Thrombocytopenia.* Immune thrombocytopenic purpura can follow viral infection, with an increased incidence of intracranial hemorrhage. Patients with thrombotic thrombocytopenic purpura have prominent neurologic symptoms including headache, hemiparesis, aphasia, and seizures. Corticosteroids and plasma exchange are of benefit in treatment.

4. *Hemophilia.* Patients with hemophilia are predisposed to develop intracranial hemorrhage, subdural hematoma, subarachnoid hemorrhage, and epidural hematoma of the spinal cord. Peripheral neuropathies may develop secondary to compression by soft-tissue hemorrhage, particularly femoral neuropathy from retroperitoneal bleeding. These bleeding complications also may occur in patients receiving anticoagulation therapy.

Note: Antiphospholipid antibodies, including lupus anticoagulant and anticardiolipin antibodies, may be associated with focal cerebral ischemia and should be tested for in young patients with unexplained cerebral ischemic events. There is a variable relationship between the presence of these antibodies and other collagen vascular disorders such as lupus. Cardiac disease (e.g., marantic endocarditis) often underlies the stroke syndromes in such patients.

PULMONARY DISEASE

1. *Respiratory insufficiency.* Hypoxia, hypercapnia, and respiratory acidosis may cause headache, mental status changes, motor disturbances, ocular abnormalities, and paresthesias.

Twitching and tremor result from increased sympathetic nervous system activity. Asterixis, generalized seizures, and myoclonus may occur. Polycythemia from chronic respiratory insufficiency causes headache and dizziness.

2. *Hyperventilation.* Anxious individuals may have neurologic symptoms including paresthesias if they hyperventilate, lightheadedness, altered consciousness, carpal spasm, muscle cramps, visual blurring, dyspnea, chest pain, and an elicitable Chvostek sign. Hyperventilation syndrome is usually psychogenic, but it may be associated with medication, alcohol withdrawal, or central nervous system (CNS) lesions. Rebreathing into a paper bag at the first awareness of symptoms and taking beta blockers may be helpful.

RHEUMATOLOGIC DISEASES, SARCOIDOSIS, AND VASCULITIDES

1. *Systemic lupus erythematosus (SLE).* Half of patients with lupus have neurologic manifestations, but most have an established diagnosis of SLE before neurologic manifestations develop. CNS lupus includes seizures, paresis, ataxia, chorea, scotomata, meningitis, cranial neuropathies, and optic neuritis. CNS lupus usually is treated with corticosteroids, cyclophosphamide, azathioprine, or plasmapheresis; CNS infections are more frequent in patients with lupus because of immunosuppressive therapy. Psychotropic medications may provide symptomatic relief of neuropsychiatric manifestations. The peripheral nervous system (PNS) is affected less frequently than the CNS, but patients may have sensory and sensorimotor neuropathies, mononeuropathies, mononeuritis multiplex, and an acute ascending sensorimotor neuropathy similar to Guillain-Barré syndrome.

2. *Sjögren's syndrome.* Neurologic manifestations of Sjögren's syndrome include seizures, movement disorders, psychiatric symptoms, aseptic meningitis, symptoms mimicking multiple sclerosis, and progressive dementia. PNS involvement (occurring in 25% of patients) includes polyneuropathy, characteristically a sensory neuropathy. Spinal cord involvement includes progressive myelopathy, transverse myelopathy, Brown-Séquard syndrome, neurogenic bladder, and spinal subarachnoid hemorrhage. Sjögren's syndrome also is

associated with neuromuscular disorders including myasthenia gravis, polymyositis, and inclusion body myositis. Treatment of CNS Sjögren's syndrome involves the use of steroids or cyclophosphamide.

3. *Rheumatoid arthritis (RA).* Neurologic manifestations of RA most often occur in patients with longstanding disease and with positive rheumatoid factor. Neuropathy is common. Compression or entrapment neuropathy occurs when swollen tissues compress peripheral nerves. Most common is median nerve compression at the wrist (carpal tunnel syndrome). Distal sensory neuropathies with dysesthesia or burning in the hands or feet occur, but these symptoms are often difficult to distinguish from the accompanying arthritis. Sensorimotor neuropathy is less common, is progressive, and can be disabling. Myelopathy also can affect patients with RA because the cervical spine frequently is involved and the cervical canal can become narrowed during neck flexion after atlantoaxial subluxation. Posterior circulation symptoms including vertigo and weakness can occur because of vertebral artery flow compromise by compression or thrombosis. Patients with advanced RA should wear cervical collars when driving or riding in a car and should have cervical spine films in flexion (provided there is no odontoid fracture) before undergoing general anesthesia. RA also may be associated with a myopathy.

4. *Osteoarthritis.* Spinal canal contents and spinal nerves may be compressed by osteoarthritis from intervertebral disc disease, spinal stenosis, and bony impingement, and peripheral nerves may become entrapped, all resulting in neurologic symptoms.

5. *Sarcoidosis.* Granulomas in the CNS can occur in extradural, subdural, leptomeningeal, and parenchymal locations, causing a wide spectrum of CNS symptoms that include (a) aseptic meningitis with headache, lethargy, vomiting, papilledema, and meningismus; (b) hydrocephalus secondary to granulomatous obstruction of cerebrospinal fluid (CSF); (c) basilar meningitis affecting cranial nerves VII through XII and the optic nerve; and (d) granulomas in the cerebral hemispheres, which can cause progressive dementia and epileptic foci. In sarcoidosis, hypercalcemia or opportunistic infections also may cause neurologic symptoms.

Occasionally, patients have a hypothalamic syndrome, which may include disturbance affecting appetite, sleep, salt and water balance, and behavior. CSF usually shows elevated protein, a mononuclear pleocytosis, and decreased glucose. Peripheral neuropathy with mononeuritis multiplex or slowly progressive symmetric sensorimotor neuropathy also is seen.

6. *Vasculitis.* CNS *vasculitis* may cause headache, behavioral changes, memory impairment, psychiatric symptoms, alteration in consciousness, and generalized seizures. Focal cerebral deficits with a strokelike picture can be caused by vasculitis and should be considered, particularly in a young patient. Cranial nerve palsies also may occur. Neurologic symptoms may be the only initial manifestation of a systemic vasculitis. *In the PNS,* mononeuritis multiplex and a distal symmetric "stocking glove" sensorimotor polyneuropathy may occur. Patients experience severe, burning dysesthetic pain in the distribution of the involved nerves. Painful focal neuropathies should suggest the possibility of vasculitis. Patients may have an elevated erythrocyte sedimentation rate and CSF protein and lymphocytic pleocytosis in the CSF during active disease. Magnetic resonance imaging (MRI) demonstrates small areas of cerebral infarction. However, a brain, meningeal, or peripheral nerve biopsy specimen is often necessary to make a definitive diagnosis of CNS or PNS vasculitis. Treatment involves removing possible inciting antigens such as medications, infectious agents, or environmental toxins. Immunosuppressive therapy with corticosteroids and cytotoxic drugs (especially cyclophosphamide) is usually helpful.

OTHER DISORDERS

1. A *reversible posterior hemisphere leukoencephalopathy* syndrome has been described in patients with several acute systemic illnesses. Symptoms include headache, altered mental function, seizures, and a striking loss of vision, accompanied by reversible white matter changes on MRI. Treatment of hypertension or removal of offending medications such as cyclosporine may hasten recovery.

2. *Organ transplantation* commonly is accompanied by neurologic disorders. These complications relate to the operation, immunosuppressive medications, infections, graft versus host, other immunologic reactions, and secondary effects of organ failure.

3. *Critical illness* is accompanied by many neurologic problems. Critical illness polyneuropathy is a syndrome in patients with long-term, complicated intensive care unit (ICU) stays who develop a severe neuropathy that causes quadriparesis and may affect respiratory muscles. The specific etiology is unknown, but sepsis is implicated in its pathogenesis. Seizures, hypoxic-ischemic disease, stroke, and metabolic encephalopathy are common and often underrecognized in the ICU. A prolonged neuromuscular paralysis sometimes is seen after the use of paralyzing agents, particularly in the presence of renal failure. Similarly, a severe myopathy sometimes is seen in the ICU after intravenous steroid therapy. Also, theophylline may precipitate subclinical status epilepticus in patients in the ICU.

Suggested Reading

Bleck TP, Smith MC, Serge J-C, et al. Neurologic complications of critical medical illness. *Crit Care Med* 1993;21:98–103.

Futrell N, Schultz LR, Millikan C. Central nervous system disease in patients with systemic lupus erythematosus. *Neurology* 1992;42:1649–1657.

Ghezzi A, Zaffaroni M. Neurological manifestations of gastrointestinal disorders, with particular reference to the differential diagnosis of multiple sclerosis. *Neurol Sci* 2001;22 (suppl 2):S117–S122.

Grant I, Hunder GG, Homburg HA, et al. Peripheral neuropathy associated with sicca complex. *Neurology* 1997;48:855–862.

Hietaharju A, YliKerttula U, Hakkinen V, et al. Nervous system manifestations in Sjögren's syndrome. *Acta Neurol Scand* 1990;81:144–152.

Hinchley J, Chaves C, Appignani B, et al. A reversible posterior leukoencephalopathy syndrome. *N Engl J Med* 1996;334:494–500.

Jozefowicz RF. Neurologic manifestations of pulmonary disease. *Neurol Clin* 1989;7:605–616.

Kaminski HJ, Ruff RL. Neurologic complications of endocrine diseases. *Neurol Clin* 1989;7:489–508.

Khamashta MA, Cuandrado MJ, Mujic F, et al. The management of thrombosis in the antiphospholipid-antibody syndrome. *N Engl J Med* 1995;332:993–997.

Lossos A, River Y, Eliakim A, et al. Neurologic aspects of inflammatory bowel disease. *Neurology* 1995;45:416–421.

Massey EW, Riggs JE. Neurologic manifestations of hematologic disease. *Neurol Clin* 1989;7:549–562.

Newman LS, Rose CS, Maier LA. Sarcoidosis. *N Engl J Med* 1997;336:1224–1234.

Patchell RA. Neurological complications of organ transplantation. *Ann Neurol* 1994;36:688–703.

Riordan SM, Williams R. Treatment of hepatic encephalopathy. *N Engl J Med* 1997;337:473–479.

Sterns RH. Neurologic sequelae after treatment of severe hyponatremia: a multicenter perspective. *J Am Soc Nephrol* 1994;4:1522–1530.

Torres CF, Moxley RT. Hypothyroid neuropathy and myopathy: clinical and electrodiagnostic longitudinal findings. *J Neurol* 1990;237:271–274.

Chapter 29

Treatment of Pain in Neurologic Disease

A working understanding of pain and its treatment is important in the management of many patients with neurologic disease. Consider the following points:

1. Pain is a subjective symptom. There are no physical findings that quantify or exclude the presence of pain. Assume that the patient has pain, and then approach management.
2. Pain can be quantified by the patient. Numerous studies have shown that a visual analog scale, in which the patient bisects a line that goes from "no pain" to "maximal pain," is the best method of quantifying pain. It is simple and provides the physician with a "semiobjective" measure of whether pain is improving or worsening.
3. Patients with chronic pain often develop depression and are misunderstood by physicians or shunned as "difficult" patients. In addition, there may be workers' compensation or litigation issues that complicate the doctor–patient relationship. The physician may develop "compassion fatigue" when dealing with a chronically disabled patient in pain. Chronic pain is often best managed in a center with comprehensive services.

TREATMENT OF PAIN

It is best to use a "stepped" approach in pain management.

1. Begin with simple analgesics such as acetaminophen, aspirin, and nonsteroidal medications.

2. Addition of a tricyclic antidepressant may be useful in chronic pain, neuropathic pain, and headache and in depressed patients with pain. Gradual titration of the medication dose usually works best. Amitriptyline, imipramine, and desipramine commonly are used. Selective serotonin reuptake inhibitors are less effective in pain management. Venlafaxine and nefazodone are antidepressants with potential efficacy in pain management.

3. Antiepileptic medication also may be used in chronic pain management, particularly when pain is neuropathic. Phenytoin, carbamazepine, valproic acid, and gabapentin each can be of benefit. Gabapentin is particularly useful in trigeminal neuralgia and in painful peripheral neuropathy. It has minimal interaction with other medications. Other newer antiepileptic medications such as lamotrigine, topiramate, and levetiracetam also are used for this indication.

4. Steroids may be used in certain situations, particularly for short-term therapy in patients with cancer.

5. Low-potency narcotic medication may be useful (e.g., codeine in combination with aspirin, acetaminophen, or propoxyphene).

6. Higher-potency narcotic medications are used when there is cancer-related pain, for short-term acute severe pain, or in a controlled program in chronic neuropathic pain. Patients who have pain and are not "drug seeking" are at low risk of addiction with such medications. The patient plays an important role in therapy and must be educated by the physician. Thus, there is no "right" dose for pain control, and the dose must be titrated with the patient's help to be most effective. Useful medications include oxycodone, morphine in various preparations, and transdermal fentanyl. In acute postoperative pain, patient-controlled analgesia with an intravenous pump is effective. Occasionally, methadone may be beneficial.

7. Providing pain medications before they are needed is better than on a demand basis. By providing the pain medication regularly, the total dose required may be lower and patient discomfort will be lessened while waiting for the next dose to take effect.

8. Topical therapies may be useful in focal pain syndromes. Capsaicin cream may be helpful with a painful joint or in dis-

tal foot pain from neuropathy. Lidocaine patches may be useful, particularly for focal pain syndromes such as postherpetic neuralgia.

9. Nonpharmacologic approaches to pain management may be helpful. These include physical measures such as warm or cold compresses, transcutaneous electrical nerve stimulation stimulators, massage therapy, chiropractic manipulation, and acupuncture; behavioral therapy such as biofeedback and relaxation therapy; and exercise and stretching programs.

10. *Surgical approaches* are used in refractory pain disorders. Surgical approaches are limited by cost and morbidity. The most common procedures include implanted pumps for baclofen or morphine for spinal cord pain and spasticity, spinal cord stimulators for refractory low back pain syndromes, thalamic stimulators for central pain syndromes, and dorsal root entry zone lesions for focal root and refractory trigeminal neuralgia.

Suggested Reading

Bonica JJ, ed. *Management of pain,* 2nd ed. Philadelphia: Lea & Febiger, 1990.

Bradley LA, McKendree-Smith NL. Central nervous system mechanisms of pain in fibromyalgia and other musculoskeletal disorders: behavioral and psychologic treatment approaches. *Curr Opin Rheumatol* 2002;14(1):45–51.

Galer BS. Neuropathic pain of peripheral origin: advances in pharmacologic treatment. *Neurology* 1995;45(suppl 9):S17–S25.

Gonzalez GR. Central pain: diagnosis and treatment strategies. *Neurology* 1995;45(suppl 9):S11–S16.

Hammack JE, Loprinzi CL. Use of orally administered opioids for cancer-related pain. *Mayo Clin Proc* 1994;69:384–390.

Max MB, Lynch SA, Muir J, et al. Effects of desipramine, amitriptyline, and fluoxetine on pain in diabetic neuropathy. *N Engl J Med* 1992; 326:1250–1256.

Rowbotham MC. Chronic pain: from theory to practical management. *Neurology* 1995;45(suppl 9):S5–S10.

Tremont-Lukats IW, Megeff C, Backonja MM. Anticonvulsants for neuropathic pain syndromes: mechanisms of action and place in therapy. *Drugs* 2000;60:1029–1052.

Wasner G, Shattschneider J, Binder A, et al. Complex regional pain syndrome—diagnostic, mechanisms, CNS involvement and therapy. *Spinal Cord* 2003;41:61–75.

Chapter 30

Lumbar Puncture and Cerebrospinal Fluid

INDICATIONS

1. When central nervous system (CNS) infection (meningitis, encephalitis) is suspected, one must examine the cerebrospinal fluid (CSF). However, there is an exception: lumbar puncture (LP) should not be performed if one suspects brain abscess or another significant space-occupying mass lesion.

2. An LP is performed to diagnose subarachnoid hemorrhage when that diagnosis is strongly suspected and the computed tomography (CT) scan result is negative.

3. An LP is done when CSF chemistries have diagnostic value (e.g., gamma globulin and oligoclonal banding in multiple sclerosis).

4. LP is needed for the study of *CSF pressure*:
   - To check for increased pressure in suspected pseudotumor cerebri
   - To check for low pressure in spontaneous intracranial hypotension headache
   - In normal pressure hydrocephalus when removal of CSF may improve gait and mentation

5. LP is done for cytology when carcinomatous or lymphomatous meningitis is suspected. Remember to take large volumes for cytology. First tap results are often negative, and a second or third tap may be required to demonstrate abnormal cells.

6. *Therapeutically*, an LP may be done to inject methotrexate or ara-c for CNS leukemia or amphotericin B for fungal menin-

gitis or to remove fluid as treatment for benign increased intracranial pressure.

CONTRAINDICATIONS

Contraindications to LP include the following:

1. Infection at the site of the LP
2. Severe thrombocytopenia or uncorrected bleeding disorder
3. When a cerebral *mass lesion* is suspected, particularly in a patient with lateralized neurologic signs or a possible mass in the posterior fossa
4. *Brain abscess* (usually seen in congenital heart disease with right-to-left shunts, otitis media, or lung disease). This may produce transtentorial or foramen magnum herniation after LP.
5. *Brain tumors.* This may lead to herniation after LP, especially when located in the posterior fossa.
6. *Subdural hematoma.* This is not usually diagnosed by LP, and the removal of fluid may be harmful.
7. *Intracranial hemorrhage.* This condition is best diagnosed by CT scan. In these instances, a CT scan or magnetic resonance imaging (MRI) for definition of the midline and a search for a mass lesion should be done before the LP.
8. *Spinal block.* This is a relative contraindication to LP; a CT scan or MRI should be done before considering an LP.
9. *Presence of papilledema* (a check of the fundi must precede each LP) without radiologic examination. An LP ultimately may be done in a patient with papilledema (e.g., in pseudo-tumor or if CSF examination is crucial) but only after neurologic or neurosurgical consultation.
10. In the presence of spinal epidural abscess. Performing an LP in this setting may spread infection to the CSF.

COMPLICATIONS

Post-LP headache occurs in 10% to 30% of patients. It is characteristically exacerbated by sitting or standing, and it is relieved by lying flat. It is seen within the first 1 to 3 days after the LP; it usually lasts 2 to 5 days, although it may persist for weeks. Treatment consists of bed rest and fluids. The mechanism of the headache is believed to be continued CSF leakage through the dural hole at the site of the LP, with subsequent intracranial traction on the meninges. Caffeinated beverages, ergot preparations, and theo-phylline may be helpful in this headache. Severe leaks can be treated by the placement of a blood patch by an anesthesiologist or neurosurgeon. Post-LP headache may be minimized by using a small-gauge needle (22 or 20), using an atraumatic LP needle, inserting the needle parallel to the dural fibers so they are spread apart rather than torn, and having the patient turn prone before removing the needle. Having the patient lie in bed after LP does not appear to reduce the incidence of post-LP headache and no longer is recommended. Patients with migraine are par-ticularly prone to post-LP headaches.

When there is an unexpected *increased opening pressure* (it must stay elevated after the patient has relaxed with legs extended and a few minutes have elapsed from the onset of the LP), remove minimal fluid needed for studies. One may leave the needle in with the stopcock closed to prevent further leak-age. Neurologic or neurosurgical consultation should be obtained, the use of mannitol or steroids should be considered, and the patient should be watched carefully over the ensuing hours for signs of deterioration. Patients with meningitis may have markedly elevated pressures, but these pressures are not as dangerous as increased intracranial pressure secondary to a focal lesion. Remember, hypercarbia, water intoxication, and hyper-tensive encephalopathy are remediable causes of increased intracranial pressure. When the intracranial pressure is increased and there is neurologic deterioration immediately or during the hours after the LP, treatment with osmotic dehydrat-ing agents and steroids is indicated (see Chapter 31).

In cryptococcal meningitis, acutely elevated CSF pressures may lead to blindness from optic nerve pressure, even when CT scan is normal. Treatment with continuous lumbar or ventricular drainage in combination with antibiotics is usually effective.

If the patient has a partial or almost complete *spinal block* sec-ondary to compression of the cord (e.g., by tumor), CSF removal may cause rapid worsening of the block. Signs of block include abnormal manometric findings and xanthochromic fluid (increased protein) under low pressure (see Chapter 9 for treat-ment).

METHOD

The puncture is carried out in the midline between the L3 to L4 or L4 to L5 interspaces located by the level of the iliac crest.

1. Insert the bevel of the needle parallel to the long axis of the spine.
2. If manometric studies and myelography are not being performed, use a 20- or 22-gauge needle.
3. Note the opening and closing pressures and the amount of fluid removed.
4. Coughing or abdominal pressure causes delayed venous return around the cord and should increase CSF flow and pressure. These maneuvers show that the needle is in place, but they do not test for spinal subarachnoid block. To do this, increase the jugular pressure (with hand pressure or a blood pressure cuff around the neck) and measure the rise and fall of CSF pressure. Manometric studies are not done routinely and are never performed if the baseline pressure is elevated or an intracranial lesion is suspected.
5. *Proper positioning* of the patient is crucial for successful LP. The patient should be placed in the fetal position with the patient's back at right angles to the bed. Insert the needle under the skin (after local anesthesia) and then decide on the angle of entry. Make sure the needle is strictly perpendicular to the patient's waist and angled toward the umbilicus. Once the needle has been advanced, if it does not enter the subarachnoid space or if it encounters bone, the direction of the needle cannot be changed. Pull the needle back to just beneath the skin and redirect it. With experience, one will learn to recognize the familiar "pop" as the needle enters the subarachnoid space. If the LP is impossible in the fetal position, have the patient sit up and lean forward grasping a pillow; try again in the sitting position (it is easier to gauge the midline). Remember, pressure measurements are difficult to interpret in the sitting position, and it may be useful to have the patient lie down after the needle is inserted. It is useful to ask the patient if the needle is off to the left or to the right. This helps the physician readjust the direction of the needle.

When an LP is impossible because of bony anomalies or local infection and CSF examination is crucial, one should arrange for a cisternal or cervical (C1–C2) tap under fluoroscopy.

EXAMINATION OF THE CEREBROSPINAL FLUID

1. *Collect four tubes* of fluid: one tube is used for cell count, one is for chemistries, one is for bacteriologic studies, and one is saved for future use (e.g., a sample may be lost, an unexpected chemistry value may require a repeat determination, or a new test may be wanted). If a traumatic tap is suspected, cells are counted in the first and fourth tubes. Some send tubes 1 and 4 for cell count with 1 mL in each and send tubes 2 and 3 for chemistries and bacteriology. To determine whether a "traumatic tap" has occurred, fluid can be spun in a centrifuge and the presence of xanthochromia can be noted. If necessary, a repeat tap can be done at a higher interspace.

2. If red blood cells (RBCs) are present, count them in the first and fourth tubes. In subarachnoid or intracranial bleeding, the amount of blood remains constant in each tube and the blood does not clot. Decreasing numbers of cells suggest a traumatic tap. After centrifugation, the CSF from a traumatic tap will be clear, whereas with true CNS bleeding the supernatant is xanthochromic if the bleeding occurred at least 2 to 4 hours previously. Finding crenated RBCs is of no distinguishing value because they appear with true bleeding and after traumatic taps.

3. Check to see if the CSF is *clear* by comparing it with water. A CSF protein level greater than 100 mg/dL usually causes the spinal fluid to look faintly yellow. Approximately 200 to 300 white blood cells (WBCs) are needed to cause CSF cloudiness. Dark CSF may be seen with metastatic melanoma and jaundice with hyperbilirubinemia; subdural hematoma may produce xanthochromia.

4. Always examine the CSF for *cells* within 1 hour after LP and preferably sooner. Normally, there should be no polymorphonuclear neutrophils (PMNs) and no more than five mononuclear cells. When looking for tumor cells, or if the nature of the WBCs in the CSF is questioned, a cytologic examination is indicated. When bacterial or tuberculous

infection is suspected, perform a Gram stain and an acid-fast stain on the centrifuged sediment. When fungal disease is a possibility, do an India ink preparation. To help reduce the cost, hold fungal cultures, India ink, and tuberculosis (TB) cultures until results of cell count, protein, and glucose are obtained. Except in immunosuppressed patients, these will be abnormal in fungal or TB meningitis.

5. When there are RBCs in the CSF and the patient has a normal complete blood count, expect approximately 1 WBC for every 700 RBCs (make further corrections for anemia). In addition, every 700 RBCs increase the protein by approximately 1mg/dL.

6. Flow cytometry may increase the identification of neoplastic cells in patients with leptomeningeal carcinomatosis or lymphomatosis. Discuss storage media and transmission with the laboratory to optimize the analysis of the spinal fluid.

INTERPRETATION

Glucose

Increased glucose levels are usually insignificant, merely reflecting systemic hyperglycemia. With changing blood glucose, CSF glucose lags blood glucose by approximately 1 hour, and the level is approximately two thirds that of blood glucose. With systemic hyperglycemia, a concomitant blood glucose determination is needed to demonstrate a relatively decreased CSF glucose (e.g., suggesting infection) that may otherwise be considered normal.

Decreased glucose levels are seen in bacterial, tuberculous, and fungal meningitis and sometimes with meningeal involvement by neoplasm or a nontuberculous granulomatous process, such as sarcoidosis. Although characteristically normal in viral infections, the CSF glucose level has been reported to be low with certain CNS viral infections (herpes, mumps, lymphocytic choriomeningitis). Decreased CSF glucose is secondary to changes in carbohydrate metabolism by neural tissue, WBC use of glucose, and alteration of glucose transport into the CNS.

Protein

Protein levels are increased in many neurologic diseases and usually reflect an abnormality in the blood–brain barrier. Elevated levels are seen in processes affecting nerve roots in peripheral neuropathy. Normal CSF protein is less than 45 mg/dL. Common processes producing increased CSF protein are as follows:

1. *Diabetes* frequently causes protein elevations (up to 150 mg/dL, or even higher when significant peripheral neuropathy is present). Look for unrecognized diabetes when there is an unexpected protein elevation. The mechanism probably is related to dorsal root ganglia involvement.

2. *Brain tumor* frequently produces protein elevations of 100 to 200 mg/100 mL, although the level may be normal. Marked increases are seen in meningiomas, acoustic neuromas, and tumors near the ventricles (e.g., ependymomas). CSF protein in brainstem gliomas is generally normal. Encapsulated *brain abscesses* produce elevations similar to those seen in brain tumors.

3. *Spinal cord tumors* also increase protein levels, often to extremely high levels (e.g., 750–1,000 mg/dL), especially when a block is present.

4. *Multiple sclerosis* may cause protein elevation in some patients, but the elevation is usually mild. Protein levels greater than 80 mg/dL in a patient with multiple sclerosis make the diagnosis suspect.

5. *Acute purulent meningitis* invariably elevates the protein level regardless of the cause, as do subacute and chronic granulomatous meningitis. Viral infections of the CNS are associated with normal protein levels or mild increases in protein initially with an increase later, which serves as a clue to the diagnosis. Carcinomatous meningitis causes significant elevation of CSF protein.

6. *Infectious polyneuritis* (Guillain-Barré syndrome) characteristically causes increased protein levels. The protein is frequently normal during the first few days of the illness but increases after 1 week.

7. *Syphilis* produces increased protein levels in the meningovascular form and general paresis; the CSF may be normal in longstanding tabes.

8. Mild to moderate elevations may be seen in myxedema, uremia, connective tissue disorders, and Cushing's disease.

9. *Cerebrovascular disease* generally causes no protein elevation or only mild increases. However, there may be large increases with cerebral hemorrhage because of serum protein in the CSF.

Gamma Globulin

The measurement of gamma globulin is used most frequently to support the diagnosis of multiple sclerosis. Normally, gamma globulin represents 13% to 15% or less of total protein. (If total protein values are less than 20 mg/100 mL, the percentage of gamma globulin may be unreliable.) Gamma globulin is elevated in multiple sclerosis, subacute sclerosing panencephalitis, Lyme disease, general paresis, herpes encephalitis, myxedema, some cases of carcinomatous cerebellar degeneration, and some connective tissue diseases (e.g., lupus). Measurement of immunoglobulin G (IgG), albumin ratio (normally less than 0.18), measurement of IgG synthesis rate, or detection of oligoclonal bands provides similar information.

Pleocytosis

PMNs in the CSF suggest a bacterial infection, and lymphocytes suggest a viral or chronic inflammatory process (although PMNs sometimes are seen at the onset of a viral infection). WBCs may be seen after subarachnoid hemorrhage, thrombosis, and at times with infectious mononucleosis. Eosinophils suggest a parasitic infection or dye reaction. Remember, many organic diseases of the CNS produce a mild pleocytosis. A thorough bacteriologic investigation must be carried out in all instances, although cells do not always represent infection. Carcinomatous meningitis tends to be accompanied by fewer than 100 cells in the CSF (more than 100 cells suggest an infectious process). T-cell and B-cell markers should be checked if the WBC count in the CSF is elevated and lymphomatous meningitis is suspected. The initial tap may be negative for tumor cells. The yield is increased on repeated cytologic examinations.

Note: If at CSF analysis the cell count, protein, and glucose are normal, it is highly unlikely that additional studies on the spinal fluid will be useful (unless it is a special consideration such as oligoclonal band determination in suspected multiple sclerosis).

CEREBROSPINAL FLUID PRESSURE

The *CSF pressure* is normally less than 200 mm H_2O with the patient lying down (or at the level of the foramen magnum in the sitting position). It is not affected by changes in systemic blood pressure but is exquisitely sensitive to changes in blood CO_2 (hyperventilation decreases intracranial pressure) and venous pressure.

1. Elevated pressures are seen in acute bacterial, fungal, and viral meningitis and meningoencephalitis.
2. Pressure elevation is frequent with tumors or other intracerebral mass lesions (e.g., abscess), although pressure may be normal despite a large tumor.
3. Pressure usually is elevated in intracerebral bleeding and in subarachnoid hemorrhage.
4. It is interesting that the pressure and protein may be increased, and there may be papilledema with polyneuritis or spinal tumor.
5. Unexplained elevated pressures may be caused by congestive heart failure, chronic obstructive pulmonary disease, hypercapnia, jugular venous obstruction, or pericardial effusion.
6. *Pseudotumor cerebri* (benign increased intracranial pressure) refers to increased pressure, as high as 400 to 600 mm H_2O, with papilledema, not associated with a mass lesion or hydrocephalus, and with an otherwise normal CSF. Causes include withdrawal from steroids, pregnancy and menarche, hypovitaminosis or hypervitaminosis A, hyperparathyroidism, tetracycline or phenothiazine administration, and venous sinus occlusion. Female patients with pseudotumor frequently are obese. Often the cause of pseudotumor cerebri is unknown. One must first rule out tumor and hydrocephalus (usually with CT scan or MRI) and then establish the diagnosis with LP. LPs alone are sometimes sufficient to decrease CSF pressure and reverse the process. Acetazolamide may be given to decrease CSF production, and then steroids are administered if necessary. Transient visual disturbances, such as blurring and dimming, are common in pseudotumor. More

severe visual difficulties, such as field defects and actual loss of vision, also can occur and warrant vigorous treatment of the increased pressure, including lumboperitoneal shunts in protracted cases. Optic nerve sheath fenestration may prevent blindness in some cases. Frequent monitoring of visual fields and of the optic nerve is warranted.

7. Patients may develop *spontaneous intracranial hypotension headache*, which is a positional headache worse with sitting and standing, similar to a post-LP headache but without an apparent cause. On LP, there is no pleocytosis but there is a low CSF pressure. MRI scanning with gadolinium shows diffuse meningeal enhancement, and there is often downward sagging of the brainstem on sagittal views. This disorder may be treated with fluids, steroids, and sometimes a blood patch. Nuclear medicine cisternography may show a dural tear in some cases.

Suggested Reading

Burgett RA, Purvin VA, Kawasaki A. Lumboperitoneal shunting for pseudotumor cerebri. *Neurology* 1997;49:734–739.

Evans RW. Complications of lumbar puncture. *Neurol Clin* 1998;16(1): 83–105.

Holdgate A, Cuthbert K. Perils and pitfalls of lumbar puncture in the emergency department. *Emerg Med* 2001;13(3):351–358.

Kuntz KM, Kokmen E, Stevens JC, et al. Post-lumbar puncture headache. *Neurology* 1992;42:1884–1889.

Radharkrishnan K, Ahlskog JE, Garrity JA, et al. Idiopathic intracranial hypertension. *Mayo Clin Proc* 1994;69:169–180.

Rando TA, Fishman RA. Spontaneous intracranial hypotension. *Neurology* 1992;42:481–487.

Chapter 31

Increased Intracranial Pressure

Increased intracranial pressure may be secondary to a focal mass lesion or more diffuse processes. *Signs* and *symptoms* include headache, nausea and vomiting, lethargy, diplopia (usually secondary to a sixth nerve palsy), transient visual obscurations, and papilledema. As intracranial pressure continues to increase, there may be bradycardia (50 to 60 beats/minute), elevation of blood pressure, increase in systolic pressure associated with lowering or slight elevation of diastolic pressure, and a slowing of the respiratory rate. This is termed the Cushing reflex; it is not specific for the diagnosis of increased intracranial pressure.

A symptom of increased intracranial pressure is headache, which is often worse in the morning or with bending over and sometimes with coughing or straining. Confusion, lethargy, and coma also may accompany increased intracranial pressure, depending on the chronicity and the cause. Papilledema, when present, is a useful sign. The presence of venous pulsations suggests a normal cerebrospinal fluid (CSF) pressure and makes it unlikely that intracranial pressure is present. On funduscopic examination, venous pulsations are best visualized where the vein turns and emerges from the optic nerve head.

HERNIATION SYNDROMES

There are three clinical syndromes of transtentorial herniation. Two represent loss of neurologic function that begins in the cerebral hemispheres and progresses to involve upper and then lower brainstem, which is fatal if untreated. The third and most uncommon consists of upward herniation of posterior fossa structures; it also can be fatal.

Lateral (Uncal) Syndrome of Herniation

1. A unilaterally dilated pupil is the first sign secondary to a mass in the middle fossa. Traditionally, it was taught that this is the result of compression of the third nerve against the incisura. However, magnetic resonance imaging (MRI) studies have shown that third nerve paresis is more commonly caused by distortion of the midbrain rather than direct third nerve compression. There is a close correlation between the degree of lateral displacement and the alteration of consciousness. A contralateral hemiplegia usually is present. Respiration and consciousness usually are unimpaired. Sometimes the ipsilateral pupil is small, rather than large, and rarely the contralateral pupil dilates before the ipsilateral one.

2. Progressive pressure increase leads to increasing stupor, a more complete third nerve palsy, and sometimes an ipsilateral hemiplegia with bilateral Babinski responses. The ipsilateral hemiparesis is secondary to tentorial pressure against the opposite cerebral peduncle (Kernohan's notch). Respiration may be normal or of the central neurogenic hyperventilation pattern. There is often decerebrate posturing (arms extended at the side with inward turning, spontaneously or when a noxious stimulus is applied). Decorticate posturing (arms flexed at the elbow "pointing" to the cortex) is not usually seen with the uncal syndrome.

3. Further pressure leads to prominent brainstem dysfunction with dilation of both pupils, loss of brainstem reflexes (e.g., absent doll's eyes, no response to ice-water calorics), ataxic respiratory patterns, and bilateral decerebrate rigidity. Treatment at this stage is rarely of benefit. MRI data suggest that most patients with acute unilateral masses have upper brainstem distortion caused predominantly by horizontal shifts at or above the tentorium.

Central Syndrome of Herniation

1. Pressure is exerted centrally on the diencephalon, rather than laterally as occurs in the lateral or uncal syndrome. The

first sign is a change in alertness or behavior. Respiration is usually normal and contains frequent sighs or yawns. There may be Cheyne-Stokes respirations. Brainstem function is intact, although pupils are small but reactive to light, and there may be roving eye movements. Bilateral hyperreflexia and Babinski responses and rigidity of the extremities are usual. With progression, there is decorticate posturing. Progression to deeper coma may be sudden and does not always follow a "rostral to caudal" pattern.

2. Involvement of upper brainstem leads to dilation of both pupils and impairment of oculocephalic and oculovestibular reflexes (i.e., absent or abnormal doll's eyes or caloric response). Central neurogenic hyperventilation often occurs, and decorticate posturing progresses to decerebrate posturing. There may be wide fluctuation in body temperature.

3. Further progression leads to loss of all brainstem function with ataxic breathing, then apnea and death.

Posterior Fossa Herniation Syndrome

1. Posterior fossa lesions may cause damage by direct compression of the brainstem and by upward herniation through the tentorial hiatus. Upward herniation from the posterior fossa obliterates the ambient cisterns and aqueduct, causing hydrocephalus with obtundation or coma.

2. Midbrain compression produces an upward gaze deficit, whereas involvement of pontine pathways may cause sixth nerve palsies, ocular bobbing, and other oculomotor signs. In addition, anisocoria (asymmetric pupils) may lead to mid-position fixed pupils. *Ocular bobbing* refers to a sudden conjugate downward deviation of the eyes, followed by a slow, upward drift. It often is seen in pontine hemorrhage with coma and quadriparesis. These syndromes can develop over hours or minutes, depending on the pathologic process. The lateral (or uncal) syndrome typically is seen secondary to space-occupying lesions, such as intracranial hemorrhage or subdural hematoma, or tumor; central herniation is seen with diffuse increased intracranial pressure (e.g., Reye's syndrome or acute hydrocephalus). The posterior syndrome occurs with posterior fossa mass lesions.

AGENTS USED IN TREATING INTRACRANIAL PRESSURE

Hyperventilation

Hyperventilation may be used in acute situations (e.g., head trauma) and often is used during neurosurgical procedures. Lowering the PCO_2 to 25 to 30 mm Hg causes vasoconstriction, reduced cerebral blood flow, an immediate reduction in intracerebral blood volume, and thus a decrease of intracranial pressure. Decreasing PCO_2 to less than 25 mm Hg may be harmful because it reduces cerebral blood flow. It is also possible that less severe degrees of hyperventilation cause ischemia. If a patient brought to the emergency ward has rapid neurologic deterioration from increased intracranial pressure, whether caused by trauma or by other intracranial processes, intubation and hyperventilation often will decrease the pressure until such agents as mannitol take effect and specific neurosurgical treatment is instituted.

Mannitol

Mannitol, an osmotic dehydrating agent, may be used. A common adult dose is 25 to 50 g initially followed by 12.5 to 25 g every 6 hours, depending on serum osmolarity. Onset of action is 15 to 30 minutes. It draws intracerebral water into the intravascular space because of its hypertonicity and, for the same reason, induces diuresis. In addition, the mechanism of action may involve changes in cerebral blood flow rheology and osmotic diuresis. It is usually not given for more than 24 to 48 hours and is used in acute situations to "buy time" (e.g., after head trauma, deterioration from an expanding intracranial process), often before neurosurgical intervention.

Urea is similar to mannitol in its use, mode of action, and dose. These agents must be given with caution to patients with renal and cardiac disease. There may be "rebound" after their use (viz., return of water intracerebrally) because small amounts cross the blood–brain barrier. Lower doses of mannitol (250 mg/kg) reduce the rebound brain edema sometimes seen with mannitol. Diuretics such as furosemide often are given as a supplement to mannitol. An osmolarity of approximately 300 to 310 mosmol/L appears to be optimal. Electrolytes and osmolarity should be checked as clinically indicated, usually every 12 hours in an acute situation.

Steroids

Steroids (e.g., dexamethasone) are used acutely and chronically [10 mg intravenously (IV) as initial bolus, then 4 to 6 mg IV, intramuscularly, or orally every 4 to 6 hours]. The onset of action is approximately 12 hours. Dexamethasone is given in acute situations and may become the mainstay of treatment after 12 to 24 hours. Dexamethasone is used to treat the vasogenic edema associated with brain tumor and abscess, after some neurosurgical procedures, and often concomitantly with radiation therapy to the brain. The mechanism of steroid action in these situations is poorly understood. Patients receiving steroids for more than a few hours usually receive cimetidine, ranitidine, or oral antacids. Steroids are probably not beneficial in treating adults with trauma-induced cerebral edema or for cytotoxic edema associated with hypoxia, cerebral infarcts, or cerebral hemorrhage.

Ventricular Drainage

Ventricular puncture and drainage may be done by a neurosurgeon when acute hydrocephalus occurs and mechanical release of increased intracranial pressure is needed. Ventricular puncture and placement of an intraventricular catheter may be done in the emergency room or in the intensive care unit. Lumbar drainage may be useful in some meningitides such as cryptococcal meningitis because an acute block of CSF flow requires artificial means to remove CSF. If untreated, blindness and coma may occur as a result of a decreased cerebral perfusion pressure (mean arterial pressure minus intracranial pressure).

Barbiturates

A controversial contribution to intracranial pressure control is the use of barbiturates. They usually are used when other attempts to decrease intracranial pressure have failed and should be used only in conjunction with an intraventricular pressure monitor in an intensive care unit. Pentobarbital is the most widely used agent. Its mechanism of action in reducing intracranial pressure is unknown.

Note: Metabolic factors such as hypoxia, hypercarbia, and hyperthermia can increase intracranial pressure. Twisted neck positions leading to kinking of the jugular veins and high mean airway pressures also can increase intracranial pressure. Hyperthermia invariably increases intracranial pressure and should be managed aggressively.

TREATMENT

When *transtentorial herniation* is in progress (see earlier), mannitol should be administered immediately and neurosurgical consultation should be obtained. This refers to trauma, abrupt changes intracerebrally secondary to a vascular event, or deterioration after LP. Concomitantly with mannitol administration, dexamethasone and furosemide should be given. If clinically appropriate, intubation and hyperventilation also are indicated.

In the *stroke patient* with a component of cerebral swelling or intracerebral hemorrhage (demonstrated by midline shift on computed tomography scan accompanying decreased level of consciousness), corticosteroids appear to be of no value. Cerebral swelling secondary to thrombosis or embolus is most pronounced approximately 48 hours after the event, whereas intracerebral hemorrhage usually increases the intracranial pressure acutely. Such measures as fluid restriction and keeping the patient's head elevated are helpful. Hyperventilation may be indicated. In some centers, small doses of mannitol (0.25 g/kg) and intracranial pressure monitoring are used. Studies suggest that hemispheric decompression with removal of the overlying skull may be life saving in certain patients with stroke and massive edema.

Patients with *brain tumors* (primary or secondary) often are treated with steroids after diagnosis, during radiation therapy, and sometimes on a chronic basis. Increased intracranial pressure caused by metastatic brain tumor tends to respond better to steroids than that caused by primary brain tumor.

Continuous monitoring of increased intracranial pressure with pressure monitoring devices is now possible and may be useful in certain patients with severe head injury or stroke. Intraventricular catheters are used most commonly and aid in therapeutic decisions.

Suggested Reading

Brazis PW, Lee AG. Elevated intracranial pressure and pseudotumor cerebri. *Curr Opin Opthalmol* 1998;9(6):27–32.

Fisher CM. Brain herniation: a revision of classical concepts. *Can J Neurol Sci* 1995;22:83–91.

Marik P, Chen K, Varon J, et al. Management of increased intracranial pressure: a review for clinicians. *J Emerg Med* 1999;17(4):711–719.

McDonald C, Carter BS. Medical management of increased intracranial pressure after spontaneous intracerebral hemorrhage. *Neurosurg Clin North Am* 2002;13(3):335–338.

Roberts I, Schierhout G, Wakai A. Mannitol for acute traumatic brain injury. *Cochrane Database Syst Rev* 2003;(2):CD001049

Ropper AH. A preliminary MRI study of the geometry of brain displacement and level of consciousness with acute intracranial masses. *Neurology* 1989;39:622–627.

Xi G, Keep RF, Hoff JT. Pathophysiology of brain edema formation. *Neurosurg Clin North Am* 2002;13(3):371–383.

Xiao F. Bench to bedside: brain edema and cerebral resuscitation: the present and the future. *Acad Emerg Med* 2002;9(9):933–946.

Chapter 32

Traumatic Brain Injury

Damage to the brain after trauma may be caused by direct injury from bone fragments or penetrating missiles; impact of brain against the base of the skull; shearing forces causing axonal injury within the white matter; or secondary phenomena such as hematomas, edema, and anoxic injury caused by respiratory difficulty. Rapid assessment and resuscitation are crucial in reducing secondary damage and preserving the potential for recovery. Head injury is a major cause of death and disability at all ages, particularly in people younger than age 25 years.

Head injury is a dynamic process. The most important parameters to monitor are the patient's level of consciousness and mental status. Following are important guidelines in dealing with the patient with head trauma.

1. In *severe head trauma,* control of airway and intravenous line placement are first priorities. One should assume that the patient has a fractured cervical spine and avoid turning the head; obtain cervical spine films in addition to skull film. Search for accompanying traumatic injury to abdominal and thoracic organs. If a patient has head injury and shock, assume that they are unrelated.

2. In obtaining the patient's *history,* establish the mode of injury and whether there was an associated anoxic period. Were there other factors such as drug and alcohol ingestion, exposure and hypothermia, or other medical problems? Patients who "talk and then deteriorate" are at high risk of harboring

an intracranial hematoma and may require immediate neurosurgical intervention.

3. All patients with head trauma require *neurologic examination,* which must include (a) careful documentation of the patient's level of consciousness and ability to carry out mental tasks, (b) a careful look at the tympanic membranes for evidence of basilar skull fracture (blood or cerebrospinal fluid), (c) scalp examination for evidence of localized areas of trauma, (d) precise recording of pupillary size and reaction, and (e) a check for hemiparesis and presence or absence of up-going toes. The Glasgow Coma Scale, a simple and reproducible scale that allows comparison of the patient's state at different times, also should be done as part of the examination (Table 32.1).

4. *Concussion* is defined as an immediate and transient loss of consciousness or other neurologic function after head injury. There may be amnesia for events before or after the amnesia (retrograde or anterograde amnesia).

5. *Observation in the hospital* for 24 to 48 hours and *neurosurgical consultation* are appropriate for a patient with any focal abnormalities on neurologic examination, unconsciousness,

TABLE 32.1. Glasgow Coma Scale

Category	Score
Eyes open	
Never	1
To pain	2
To verbal stimuli	3
Spontaneously	4
Best verbal response	
None	1
Incomprehensible	2
Inappropriate words	3
Disoriented, conversing	4
Oriented, conversing	5
Best motor response	
None	1
Extension	2
Flexion abnormal	3
Flexion withdrawal	4
Localizing pain	5
Obeys commands	6
Total	15

abnormal mental status, skull fracture, intracranial abnormalities on computed tomography (CT), or head trauma that is thought to be significant despite a normal examination. The decision to hospitalize or send a patient home who has not been unconscious and who has a normal neurologic examination may be made after careful consideration of the severity of trauma and of who will look after and monitor the patient at home.

6. One of the most feared complications of head injury is the development of an acute *subdural or epidural hematoma*, which then may cause herniation (see Chapter 31) and fatal brainstem compression. Clinically, this process manifests itself as headache; decreased level of consciousness; and, late in the course, a dilated pupil that is usually on the side of the hematoma, secondary to pressure on the third nerve. *Epidural hematoma* most commonly represents arterial bleeding secondary to tearing the middle meningeal artery on the undersurface of the temporal bone. The patient steadily may deteriorate after the trauma or experience a "lucid interval" only to deteriorate later. Most patients will have a fracture over the groove of the middle meningeal artery. *Subdural hematoma* is secondary to venous or arterial bleeding and also has the potential for brainstem compression. Subdural and epidural hematomas are diagnosed by CT scan or magnetic resonance imaging (MRI). *Chronic subdural hematomas* can present days or weeks after trauma, often in the elderly, and may cause slow behavioral changes, gait disturbances, headache, and incontinence.

7. Aside from the asymptomatic patient with no or very brief loss of consciousness, all patients should undergo CT scanning. Skull radiographs are not useful in most head injuries and will miss many significant intracranial abnormalities. They will show linear skull fractures or air fluid levels in the sinuses. CT scanning is helpful in assessing the type and severity of immediate injury, the presence of hematomas and edema, and the need for neurosurgical intervention.

8. MRI is a more sensitive modality for traumatic brain injury but often cannot be performed early in the patient's course because of neurologic, hematologic, or spinal instability. It occasionally may pick up subacute or chronic subdural hematomas missed by CT scanning.

9. All patients with severe head injuries (Glasgow Coma Scale score of 8 or less) or major skull fractures require the early attention of a neurosurgeon. Deterioration in level of consciousness, intracranial hemorrhage, or focal neurologic findings demand immediate neurosurgical assessment.

10. If the patient is deteriorating, assume intracranial pressure is increased, administer mannitol and Lasix, and obtain a CT scan rapidly.

11. The value of *prophylactic antiepileptic drugs* after traumatic brain injury is unclear. Although phenytoin may decrease seizures in the first week after head injury, it may not decrease seizures over a longer period. With penetrating injuries or major hematoma, the risk of seizures is greater, suggesting that this group of patients is better suited for prophylactic therapy.

12. The *postconcussion syndrome* includes headache, dizziness, fatigue, decreased concentration, memory disorder, irritability, depression, and other psychologic symptoms. In patients with such symptoms, medication (antidepressants) and rehabilitation may be helpful. Such patients may be difficult to treat if there are complicating social and litigation factors.

13. Although traumatic subarachnoid hemorrhage is common, lumbar puncture has no value in the patient with acute head injury and is potentially dangerous.

14. In some patients with persistent coma and a normal CT scan, diffuse axonal injury (DAI) is present. In these cases, shearing injury to axons is present. Coma of 6 to 24 hours duration is termed mild DAI, and coma of more than 24 hours is considered moderate to severe DAI, depending on the presence of brainstem signs. DAI is the most important cause of persistent disability after traumatic brain injury.

Suggested Reading

Alexander MP. A sensible approach to mild traumatic brain injury. *Neurology* 1995;45:1253–1260.

Cushman JG, Agarwal N, Fabian TC, et al. Practice management guidelines for the management of mild traumatic brain injury: the EAST practice management guidelines work group. *J Trauma* 2001;51(5): 1016–1026.

Ghajar J. Traumatic brain injury. *Lancet* 2000;356:923–929.

Gupta AK. Monitoring the injured brain in the intensive care unit. *J Postgrad Med* 2002;48(3):218–225.

Hammoud DA, Wasserman BA. Diffuse axonal injuries: pathophysiology and imaging. *Neuroimaging Clin N Am* 2002;12(2):205–216.

Marion DW, Penrod LE, Kelsey SF, et al. Treatment of traumatic brain injury with moderate hypothermia. *N Engl J Med* 1997;336:540–546.

Mazzola CA, Adelson PD. Critical care management of head trauma in children. *Crit Care Med* 2002;30(11 Suppl):S393–S401.

McDonald BC, Flashman LA, Saykin AJ. Executive dysfunction following traumatic brain injury: neural substrates and treatment strategies. *Neurorehabilitation* 2002;17(4):333–344.

McNaughton H, Harwood M. Traumatic brain injury: assessment and management. *Hosp Med* 2002;63(1):8–11.

Royo NC, Shimizu S, Schouten JW, et al. Pharmacology of traumatic brain injury. *Curr Opin Pharmacol* 2003;3(1):27–32.

Stuss DT. A sensible approach to mild traumatic brain injury. *Neurology* 1995;45:1251–1252.

Zee CS, Hovanessian A, Go JL, et al. Imaging of sequelae of head trauma. *Neuroimaging Clin N Am* 2002;12(2):325–338.

Zink BJ. Traumatic brain injury outcome: current concepts for emergency care. *Ann Emerg Med* 2001;37(3):318–332.

Chapter 33

Neurodiagnostic Procedures

ELECTROENCEPHALOGRAM

The electroencephalogram (EEG) is a physiologic monitor of cerebral cortical function. It measures electrical activity that is generated in the cerebral cortex and then synchronized and modulated by thalamic and reticular activating structures. It is primarily a measure of grey matter or neuronal function and is abnormal when there is disease affecting neurons or grey matter. Diseases of the white matter may cause slowing of the EEG as well. EEG is most useful in seizure disorders, encephalopathies, and coma.

1. *Seizure disorders.* The EEG is a key test for the diagnosis and management of patients with seizure disorders. It should be emphasized that not all patients with clinically definite seizure disorders have abnormalities on EEG and, conversely, paroxysmal EEG abnormalities sometimes are seen in people without seizure disorders. During a tonic-clonic seizure, an EEG usually demonstrates widespread electrical discharges. Complex partial seizures may show a focal buildup of rhythmic waves, and simple partial seizures may not show abnormalities on the surface EEG at all. Interictal EEGs in patients with seizure disorders are abnormal in approximately 70% of patients. Certain seizure disorders are classified according to EEG patterns:

   a. *Absence seizure,* a seizure characterized by brief losses of consciousness (e.g., staring spells of no more than several seconds), occurs almost exclusively in people between the ages of 5 and 18. It shows classic three-per-second spike-

and-wave discharges. The diagnosis of absence seizures depends on this EEG finding.

b. *Temporal lobe epilepsy* is characterized by focal EEG abnormalities in either or both temporal lobes, including sharp waves or spike discharges. These abnormalities may not be apparent on routine interictal EEGs but usually can be demonstrated by sleep EEGs or by using special scalp leads over the temporal regions. If temporal lobe epilepsy is suspected, such procedures should be carried out. Continuous monitoring may be necessary in difficult cases.

c. *Lennox-Gastaut syndrome* is a childhood syndrome, often with mental retardation, in which patients have several seizure types. The interictal EEG shows characteristic slow spike-and-wave discharges. *West syndrome* is associated with early childhood seizures called infantile spasms and has a characteristic EEG pattern of high-voltage slow waves and spikes (hypsarrhythmia).

d. Anticonvulsant medications usually do not affect the EEG, although certain medications cause specific EEG patterns (e.g., barbiturates and benzodiazepines cause beta or fast wave patterns). The EEG is often useful in the decision of whether to discontinue anticonvulsant medication (see Chapter 20).

2. *Cerebrovascular disease.* The EEG seldom is used in cerebrovascular disease. The EEG may clarify a clinical suspicion of stroke when the initial computed tomography (CT) scan is normal early in the course. In some patients with large strokes and encephalopathy, EEG may show seizure discharges.

3. *Encephalopathy.* Patients with metabolic encephalopathy of any cause have abnormal EEGs, consisting of nonfocal slowing of the EEG pattern or rhythmic bursts of symmetric frontal slowing. The EEG can be useful in identifying metabolic encephalopathies or in ruling out metabolic encephalopathies in patients with altered mental status. Sometimes these patterns can be helpful (e.g., the "triphasic" waves of hepatic encephalopathy).

4. *Coma.* For patients in a coma, the EEG can assist with identifying severe injury, subclinical seizure activity, or major asymmetries and may provide good prognostic signs such as the presence of reactivity and sleep potentials.

5. *Tumors.* Depending on the location and size of a tumor, the EEG is often abnormal, with focal slowing or spike discharges. New onset of seizures in middle age is often the presenting symptom of tumor. However, the CT scan or magnetic resonance imaging (MRI) is the major test used to diagnose tumors or other space-occupying lesions.

6. *Other diseases.* Some disorders have characteristic EEG findings (e.g., Creutzfeldt-Jakob disease, herpes simplex encephalitis, subacute sclerosing panencephalitis). Some infectious disorders of the central nervous system (CNS) do not affect brain waves (e.g., cryptococcal meningitis). Psychiatric diseases (affective disorders, schizophrenia) usually have no effect on the EEG. Migraine headaches may be associated with focal slowing. The EEG often is used as an adjunct in the diagnosis of brain death (isoelectric EEG).

Note: In selected cases, more prolonged EEG testing in combination with video monitoring, sometimes with subdural or intracerebral electrode placement, is used to localize seizure foci. This is to define whether unusual spells are indeed seizures or to localize seizures preparatory to seizure surgery. Such testing is best done in a specialized setting. Ambulatory EEG monitoring (analogous to Holter EEG) may be useful in detecting paroxysmal abnormalities, such as seizure discharges, not seen on individual EEG recordings.

ELECTROMYOGRAPHY

The electromyogram (EMG) is an electrical test measuring physiologic function in muscle. It is used to help diagnose muscle disease, disease of the neuromuscular junction, and denervation of muscles secondary to nerve or root lesions. Specific abnormalities seen in EMG include alteration of the motor unit (increased size and duration in chronic denervation), fibrillation and positive sharp waves in acute denervation, and abnormal electrical excitability in metabolic disorders.

1. Patients with *myopathy* often show certain features: (a) low-amplitude, short-duration motor unit potentials; (b) complex polyphasic motor unit potentials; and (c) increased insertional activity (e.g., bizarre high-frequency discharges). It is usually impossible to distinguish one myopathy from

another by EMG. Some myopathies (e.g., polymyositis and muscular dystrophies) may show fibrillation potentials.

2. *Myotonia* presents a characteristic pattern of hyperexcitability with persistent waxing and waning and repetitive discharges, which sound like a "dive bomber." The dive bomber pattern is not diagnostic of any single myotonic disorder.

3. Presynaptic *neuromuscular junction (NMJ) disorders* (e.g., botulism, Eaton-Lambert syndrome) may be characterized by progressive enhancement of motor unit action potentials evoked by repetitive stimulation of the motor nerve. Most also show normal amplitude miniature end-plate potentials. By contrast, postsynaptic NMJ disorders (e.g., myasthenia gravis) show a decremental response of the muscle action potential with repetitive nerve stimulation and subnormal amplitudes of the miniature endplate potentials. Both presynaptic and postsynaptic NMJ disorders show increased jitter or variation in latency between a nerve stimulus and the resulting muscle action potentials on single-fiber EMG testing.

4. *Denervation* produces increased polyphasic action potentials, bizarre high-frequency discharges, fibrillations, positive sharp waves, and fasciculations. Fibrillation potentials develop 3 to 4 weeks after the onset of nerve injury. Thus, someone with an acute root or nerve lesion may not show muscle fibrillation. Examination of muscle groups in the legs or arms may help to diagnose specific root lesions and whether denervated muscles are referable to a single root. Similarly, denervation can be used to help diagnose amyotrophic lateral sclerosis or other anterior horn cell diseases.

NERVE CONDUCTION STUDIES

Nerve conduction studies yield information about the integrity of myelin and axon in peripheral nerve. If nerve conduction studies are abnormal in all limbs, a *generalized* neuropathy is implied (e.g., diabetic or alcoholic neuropathies). Disorders that primarily affect myelin (e.g., Guillain-Barré syndrome) cause nerve conduction slowing out of proportion to EMG changes, whereas "axonal" neuropathies (e.g., caused by alcohol) cause EMG changes of denervation out of proportion to nerve conduction abnormalities. Individual nerve abnormalities can be seen in nerve entrapments (e.g., carpal tunnel) or nerve infarction or damage (e.g., mononeuritis multiplex). Nerve conduction studies are useful in focal entrapment syndromes such as carpal tunnel syndrome and ulnar entrapment at the elbow. Disorders of the proximal nerve, including the cell body, will prolong the "F response," which is a peripherally recorded potential produced by retrograde conduction of a stimulated action potential to the soma, with subsequent orthograde conduction back to the periphery. The Hoffman, or H, reflex is an orthograde motor potential generated by stimulating sensory fibers in the stretch reflex arc. Thus, an H reflex can be used to detect sensory or motor root lesions. The "F response" is particularly useful in disorders that primarily affect the proximal nerve (e.g., early stages of Guillain-Barré syndrome).

EVOKED POTENTIALS

An evoked potential is an electrical response recorded from the CNS and elicited by an external stimulus, either visual, auditory, or somatosensory. Evoked potentials are useful in localizing subtle sensory lesions and in detecting unsuspected *subclinical* sensory deficits. With the advent of MRI scanning, the use of evoked potentials has diminished.

1. *Visual evoked responses* (VERs), measured over the occiput, are stimulated by shifting checkerboard patterns in the visual fields. They are most helpful in demonstrating lesions in the optic nerves and are particularly useful in diagnosis of multiple sclerosis (MS). Most patients with a history of optic neuritis or MS have VER abnormalities. VER changes are also seen in toxic and nutritional amblyopias, tumors compressing the anterior visual pathways, Friedreich's ataxia, and pernicious anemia. VERs also may be of benefit in patients suspected of hysterical visual loss. VERs are helpful in monitoring optic nerve and chiasm function in patients with pituitary tumors or pseudotumor cerebri.

2. *Brainstem auditory evoked responses* are elicited by delivering click stimuli to either ear. Their major advantage is the ability to localize auditory pathway lesions to eighth nerve, cochlear nucleus, superior olive, lateral lemniscus, or inferior colliculus. They are exquisitely sensitive to extrinsic lesions, such as acoustic neuromas, and may detect these

lesions before they are visible by CT scan. They are also sensitive to intrinsic brainstem lesions involving the auditory pathways as seen in MS, brainstem glioma, brainstem infarcts, and olivopontocerebellar degeneration. Because they are not abolished by high doses of anesthesia or barbiturates, they are useful monitors of brainstem integrity in patients rendered comatose or treated with these agents. They may prove useful as prognostic indicators in the patient who is comatose, especially after head trauma.

3. *Somatosensory evoked responses* (SERs) are elicited by stimulating large-fiber sensory systems peripherally. Tibial and peroneal evoked responses may help to localize lesions to their respective peripheral nerves, lumbosacral plexus, dorsal spinal cord, spinomedullary junction, brainstem, and thalamus. Median nerve SERs will assess function along the arm and centrally through spinomedullary junction, brainstem, and thalamus. Pudendal SERs help to detect deficits of sensory innervation of the genitalia. Virtually any lesion compromising conduction in these systems (e.g., MS, spinal cord tumors, severe cervical spondylosis) may produce SER abnormalities. SERs are useful adjuncts to monitor spinal cord function during cord surgery.

MAGNETIC RESONANCE IMAGING

Magnetic resonance imaging (MRI) is the imaging modality of choice for several neurologic disorders, including congenital anomalies, especially those involving the posterior fossa (e.g., Arnold-Chiari); pathology of the sella turcica, including pituitary tumors; lesions involving the internal auditory canal (e.g., acoustic neuroma); lesions of the posterior fossa, including brainstem and cerebellum (e.g., brainstem gliomas, cerebellar astrocytoma); lesions of temporal lobes and white matter diseases, especially those of demyelinating origin (e.g., MS); and spinal cord lesion (e.g., spinal cord tumors, syringomyelia). MRI has become an important part of the diagnosis of stroke and is used in refractory epilepsies to assess for cortical abnormalities.

An MRI scan takes approximately 30 to 60 minutes, and during most of this time, the patient must lie motionless. If this is impossible, sedation may be required. A scan consists of a pulsating magnetic field (heard as banging sounds by the patient) and a continuous high-strength magnetic field (which the patient does not feel). An MRI cannot be performed in patients with pacemakers, intracranial aneurysm clips, or a metallic foreign body in the eye or brain.

The areas of the nervous system where MRI has a particular advantage over CT are those where there is significant bony artifact (especially brainstem and spinal cord). MRI continues to have limitations when poor patient cooperation and movement precludes a prolonged period with the patient still in the study or when the issue is deciding whether acute hemorrhage has occurred (e.g., subarachnoid hemorrhage). Advances in software and in altering pulse sequences may resolve these problems in the future.

Points of particular interest with respect to MRI imaging of the nervous system include the following:

1. *Neuroanatomy.* MRI provides a unique opportunity to visualize the neuroanatomy involved in normal and abnormal function of the nervous system. Thus, the components of the pyramidal and extrapyramidal motor system; the sensory system of the face and body; and the visual, hearing, and olfactory systems can be visualized easily in three planes. House officers and students are urged to use MRI as a valuable tool to enhance their knowledge of functional neuroanatomy and to identify the lesions and structures involved in the disease processes encountered.

2. *Seizures.* MRI is the imaging modality of choice in the evaluation of patients with new-onset seizures. Reasons for its superiority over CT in this clinical problem include the following:
   a. Its ability to image in three planes makes it more sensitive in detecting lesions that may cause seizures and in delineating their size and location. The coronal views are particularly valuable in detecting temporal lobe lesions.
   b. Seizures may be caused by arteriovenous malformations (AVMs), which are imaged well by MRI without the necessity for intravenous contrast injection.
   c. Neoplasms, either primary or secondary, may be responsible for seizures, and MRI is extremely sensitive for detecting the presence of tumors. Edema surrounding tumor is well seen with MRI.

d. Areas of abnormal brain development, particularly where grey matter movement from the germinal layer to the cortex, may be shown on MRI because of its excellent grey–white discrimination.

3. *Headaches.* MRI is valuable in the evaluation of patients with new-onset or progressive headaches because of its ability to detect brain tumor, AVM, cerebral venous thrombosis, subdural hematomas, aneurysms, or hydrocephalus.

4. *Stroke.* CT remains the imaging modality of choice in the setting of acute stroke to exclude the presence of hemorrhage. MRI is more sensitive than CT (a) in the subacute stage to detect subtle hemorrhage; (b) in imaging small infarctions, especially within the first 48 hours after symptom onset; (c) in detecting infarctions in the posterior fossa; (d) in detecting other lesions masquerading as stroke, such as brain tumor; and (e) in detecting cavernous sinus thrombosis. Techniques such as diffusion MRI and perfusion MRI can show stroke evolution within an hour of stroke onset and may give information about the viability of the injured brain areas.

5. *Head trauma.* CT remains the appropriate study in the acute evaluation of the trauma patient in searching for an extraaxial blood clot or assessing acute brain damage and acute skull injury using bone windows. MRI is preferred in the subacute state to detect extraaxial hematoma, contusion, and shearing injury.

6. *Ataxia/deafness/vertigo.* MRI is preferred over CT in evaluating the posterior fossa because, unlike with CT scanning, there are no bony artifacts. It is particularly valuable in imaging cerebellar neoplasms (astrocytoma, medulloblastoma), neoplasms of the brainstem, and acoustic neuromas or other lesions in the cerebellopontine angle.

7. *Dementia.* MRI is valuable in evaluation of the patient with dementia because of its ability to detect and delineate tumors, subdural hematoma, multiple infarcts, and cerebral atrophy.

8. *Multiple sclerosis.* MRI is useful in demonstrating the demyelinating lesions of MS. Patients without clinical evidence of brain involvement (e.g., when presenting with optic neuritis or a spinal cord lesion) frequently are found to have charac-

teristic periventricular lesions on MRI. Gadolinium enhancement shows plaques are active and may influence treatment decisions.

9. *Spine and spinal cord.* MRI is the imaging examination of choice for disorders that affect the spine or spinal cord. It is of particular value for visualizing primary spinal cord tumors (e.g., gliomas), intradural or extradural processes dial impinge on the spinal cord (e.g., meningiomas, metastatic tumors), syringomyelia, hematomyelia, and spinal stenosis. Its role in relation to CT and myelography in evaluating cervical and lumbar disc disease still is being defined, but it is already playing a major role in evaluating these processes.

10. *Amenorrhea/galactorrhea.* These symptoms may be caused by a pituitary microadenoma. The sensitivity of MRI in detecting pituitary microadenomas is equal to or greater than contrast-enhanced direct coronal thin-section CT. MRI is superior in delineating invasion of local structures (e.g., cavernous sinus) by macroadenomas.

11. *Congenital anomalies.* MRI is an excellent modality to demonstrate congenital anomalies, such as Dandy-Walker cyst in the posterior fossa, Arnold-Chiari malformation, and agenesis of the corpus callosum. It provides details of abnormal morphology in the dysmorphic brain (e.g., in derangements of myelination).

The use of paramagnetic contrast media as an adjunct to MRI further enhances the value of MRI in certain situations. These include searching for brain and leptomeningeal metastases, assessing the activity of MS plaques, and assessing for acoustic neuroma. In addition, magnetic resonance angiography (MRA) has increased the ability of MRI to assess extracranial and intracranial vessels for anomalies, aneurysms, and areas of stenosis. Magnetic resonance spectroscopy is useful in the diagnosis of brain tumors and in some metabolic disorders of the brain. Newer techniques such as diffusion tensor imaging may be beneficial in assessing the extent of cerebral edema associated with brain tumors. Functional MRI helps in showing the area of cortical activation when the patient performs a clinical task (such as moving the hand or talking). This has been helpful in assessing cortical function preoperatively when surgery must be performed near eloquent areas of the brain.

MAGNETIC RESONANCE ANGIOGRAPHY

Magnetic resonance angiography (MRA) is a technique that noninvasively images the blood vessels. The flow void seen in blood vessels is reconstructed, allowing an evaluation of the intracranial and extracranial vessels. MRA is limited in that the image may be degraded by movement and by tortuous flow in vessels, which will show up as a gap in magnetic resonance signal. However, MRA helps assess vessel stenosis, large aneurysms, AVMs, and venous sinus disease.

COMPUTED TOMOGRAPHY SCAN

Computerized axial tomography heralded a revolution in the diagnosis and management of neurologic disease. Its use lessened with the development of MRI but has reemerged with the advent of CT angiography.

Contrast enhancement in CT scanning generally is used to assist diagnosis of certain infections and tumors. The danger of "routine" contrast use relates to allergy to the dye and the effect of dye on renal function. The decision to use contrast rests on the clinical circumstances. Contrast should be avoided in patients with marginal renal function and should be used with caution in dehydrated patients with diabetes because of the risk of renal failure.

1. *Cerebrovascular disease.* The basic value of the CT scan in cerebrovascular disease is to differentiate hemorrhage from infarction. Virtually all hemorrhages show up as increased density on CT scans, whereas either no abnormality or decreased density is seen with infarction. This distinction is particularly important because it is impossible to distinguish infarction from hemorrhage on clinical grounds alone. *No patient should be anticoagulated without prior CT scan to rule out bleeding.* Of infarcts, 15% to 20% are apparent immediately on CT scan, and most moderate-sized infarcts are apparent at 3 to 5 days. The diagnosis of multiple infarcts caused by emboli also can be made by CT scan, including infarcts seen in areas that have not declared themselves clinically. CT scan can identify AVMs and aneurysms, although the precise diagnosis of these disorders usually requires arteriography.

2. *Tumors.* Virtually all tumors larger than 2 to 4 mm can be seen on CT scan. Depending on the pattern, certain diagnostic interpretations can be made. CT scan sensitivity to tumors is enhanced by perfusion with iodinated contrast agents.

3. *Hydrocephalus.* Although CT scan and MRI are useful for the demonstration of hydrocephalus, MRI is more accurate in determining the cause (e.g., aqueductal stenosis).

4. *Degenerative disease.* Patients with CNS degenerative diseases, such as Alzheimer's disease, usually have normal CT scan early in the disease. However, as patients get older, they usually have widened sulci and enlarged ventricles because of loss of brain tissue. Brain atrophy does not necessarily correlate with dementia and also can be seen in "normal" people. There are patients with degenerative disease or dementia who have normal-appearing CT scans.

5. *Subdural hematoma.* Approximately 80% of subdural hematomas, both unilateral and bilateral, can be seen on CT scan. Some subdurals may be isodense and not visualized by CT scan. These may be seen with contrast injection or with MRI scanning.

6. *Brainstem and spinal cord.* In general, the brainstem and spinal cord are better visualized on MRI than CT scan. Disease of neural foramina (e.g., disc and bony disease) is better evaluated by CT than by MRI. CT scanning is limited because one cannot image the entire spinal cord in horizontal sections. Thus, spinal CT scans should be reserved for clinical situations in which the examination suggests abnormality at a specific spinal level.

7. *Trauma.* CT is effective in differentiating many consequences of trauma in the nervous system, including fractures, epidural and subdural hematomas, and shifts of intracranial contents. CT scanning is an excellent screening method for showing intracranial shifts before performing LP.

8. CT angiography is a technique using computerized timing of injected dye to image the aortic arch, the carotids, and the intracranial structures. It may be used as a rapid method to analyze the vascular system and is being used to assess patients with acute cerebral infarction.

ARTERIOGRAPHY

Cerebral arteriography is used to define vascular disease of intracranial and extracranial vessels (e.g., carotid artery disease, AVM, and aneurysms) when less invasive procedures are inconclusive. MRA obviates the need for arteriography in many cases. For some diseases, such as the evaluation of small berry aneurysms and cerebral vasculitis, angiography remains more sensitive than MRA. Risks of arteriography include reaction to the contrast media, thrombosis or hemorrhage at the catheter introduction site, arrhythmia, transient global amnesia, seizure, and stroke. The risks of arteriography must be weighed against the benefits, particularly with the variety of alternative noninvasive procedures that are available.

Suggested Reading

Bakshi R, Lindsay BD, Kinkel PR. Brain magnetic resonance imaging in clinical neurology. In: Joynt RJ, Griggs RC, eds. *Baker's clinical neurology.* Philadelphia: Lippincott Williams & Wilkins, 1997;1:1–203.

Caruso G, Eisen A, Stalberg E, et al. Clinical EMG and glossary of terms most commonly used by clinical electromyographers. The international federation of clinical neurophysiology. *EEG Clin Neurophysiol* 1999;Suppl.52:189–198.

Flink R, Pedersen B, Guekht AB, et al. Guidelines for the use of EEG methodology in the diagnosis of epilepsy. *Acta Neurol Scand* 2002; 106(1):1–7.

Gronseth GS, Ashman EJ. Practice parameter: the usefulness of evoked potentials in identifying clinically silent lesions in patients with suspected multiple sclerosis (An evidence-based review): Report of the Quality Standards Subcommittee of the American Academy of Neurology. *Neurology* 2000:54(9):1720–1725.

Practice parameter for electrodiagnostic studies in carpal tunnel syndrome: summary statement. *Muscle Nerve* 2002;25(6):918–922.

Nederkoorn PJ, Elgersma OE, Van Der Graaf Y, et al. Carotid artery stenosis: accuracy of contrast-enhanced MR angiography for diagnosis. *Radiology* 2003 Jul 17 [Epub ahead of print] full text at radiology.rsnajhls.org.

Wechsler LR, Babikian VL. Transcranial doppler sonography. *Arch Neurol* 1994;51:1054–1059.

Chapter 34

Key Points in Neuroanatomy

The examination of the nervous system depends on knowledge of the anatomy, which underlies the clinical findings. Following are some key points of neuroanatomy to help localize and diagnose neurologic disorders.

The cerebral cortex is comprised of four lobes for each hemisphere and each lobe has specialized functions (Fig. 34.1).

1. *Frontal* lobes participate in speech (Broca's area for speech is in the dominant hemisphere), movement (corticospinal tracts originate here), personality, and initiative. Frontal eye fields participate in conjugate eye deviation, so that lesions on one side cause the eye to deviate to the ipsilateral side.

2. *Temporal* lobes participate in memory functions and auditory processing. For language, it is the dominant hemisphere; for music, it is usually the nondominant hemisphere. A unilateral temporal lesion may cause a contralateral superior quadrantanopsia as a result of involvement of optic radiations.

3. *Parietal* cortex participates in sensation, thus contralateral loss of cortical sensation occurs with lesions (two-point discrimination, identification of objects or numbers drawn in the hand). A mild hemiparesis may occur with parietal injury. Alexia, agraphia, left/right discrimination difficulty, and finger naming difficulty occur with a lesion in the left angular gyrus of the parietal lobe. Nondominant parietal lesions may cause visuospatial difficulty, dressing apraxia, a loss of awareness of the left side of the body, and topographic memory loss.

CEREBRAL CORTEX

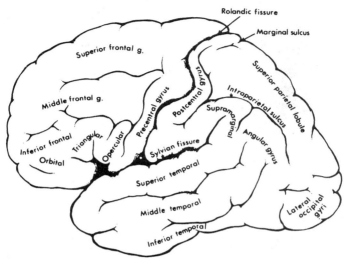

FIGURE 34.1. Left hemisphere showing frontal, parietal, temporal, and occipital lobes. (Reproduced with permission of Ms. Linda Wilson-Pauwels and B. C. Decker, Inc., Hamilton, Ontario, Canada.)

4. *Occipital* lobes participate in vision. Lesions of the occipital lobe cause visual field loss, hallucinosis, or blindness. Altered recognition of objects or faces by sight also may occur.

CIRCLE OF WILLIS

The anterior, middle, and posterior cerebral arteries supply the anteromesial cortex; the lateral frontal, temporal, and parietal lobes; and the occipital lobes, respectively. The superior cerebellar artery supplies the superior aspect of the cerebellum. The basilar artery supplies the upper brainstem, and the vertebral arteries supply the lower brainstem and cerebellum. The anastomotic circle of Willis connects the anterior and posterior circulation through the posterior communicating arteries and the left and right circulations through the anterior communicating artery. The circle of Willis is frequently anatomically incomplete (Fig. 34.2).

Circle of Willis

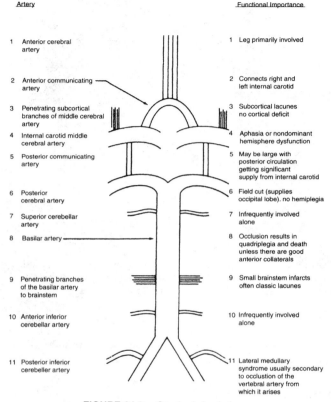

Artery	Functional Importance
1 Anterior cerebral artery	1 Leg primarily involved
2 Anterior communicating artery	2 Connects right and left internal carotid
3 Penetrating subcortical branches of middle cerebral artery	3 Subcortical lacunes no cortical deficit
4 Internal carotid middle cerebral artery	4 Aphasia or nondominant hemisphere dysfunction
5 Posterior communicating artery	5 May be large with posterior circulation getting significant supply from internal carotid
6 Posterior cerebral artery	6 Field cut (supplies occipital lobe). no hemiplegia
7 Superior cerebellar artery	7 Infrequently involved alone
8 Basilar artery	8 Occlusion results in quadriplegia and death unless there are good anterior collaterals
9 Penetrating branches of the basilar artery to brainstem	9 Small brainstem infarcts often classic lacunes
10 Anterior inferior cerebellar artery	10 Infrequently involved alone
11 Posterior inferior cerebeller artery	11 Lateral medullary syndrome usually secondary to occlusion of the vertebral artery from which it arises

FIGURE 34.2. Cerebral circulation.

The frontal eye fields exert a major influence on horizontal eye movement, each field being concerned with contralateral eye deviation. Thus, the right field causes eyes to move to the left. (The fibers cross in the pons and connect there to the extraocular muscles via the medial longitudinal fasciculus.) Both fields are constantly active, striking a balance; thus, when one is more or less active than the other, horizontal eye deviation results (Fig. 34.3).

EYE DEVIATION IN NEUROLOGIC DISEASE

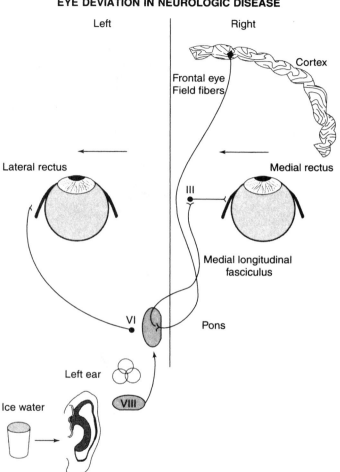

FIGURE 34.3.   In the comatose patient with an intact brainstem, ice water in the left ear causes deviation of the eyes to the left. In the patient who is awake, this deviation is counteracted voluntarily, producing nystagmus to the right.

EYE DEVIATION IN NEUROLOGIC DISEASE

Horizontal eye movements are subserved by the medial (third nerve) and lateral (sixth nerve) rectus muscles (Fig. 34.4). Inputs from the cortex and eighth nerve nuclei affect the paramedian pontine reticular formation, which drives the sixth nerve nucleus. This stimulates the ipsilateral lateral rectus and contralateral medial rectus, connecting with the latter through the medial longitudinal fasciculus. A lesion in the sixth nerve nucleus causes a paralysis of ipsilateral gaze (cannot bring the eyes to the side injured because of weakness in the ipsilateral lateral rectus and contralateral medial rectus).

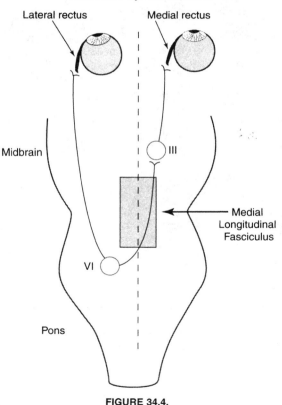

Horizontal Eye Movements

FIGURE 34.4.

Horizontal Eye Movements

A *destructive lesion* in the hemisphere or subcortex causes eyes to deviate toward the same side as the lesion. Thus, with a right-sided lesion, the eyes are deviated to the right. An *excitatory lesion* at the cortical level (e.g., a seizure) causes eyes to deviate to the contralateral side. A *destructive lesion* in the pons causes eyes to deviate to the side opposite the damage. Thus, with a left-sided lesion, eyes deviate to the right. Eye deviation secondary to hemisphere lesions, but not brainstem lesions, may be overcome by brainstem reflexes (e.g., doll's eyes maneuver).

Visual Pathways (Fig. 34.5)

1. *Blindness in one eye* represents retinal or ipsilateral optic nerve dysfunction. The optic nerve frequently is involved in multiple sclerosis (optic neuritis), producing unilateral blindness; it also may be involved by tumor (optic glioma) or undergo

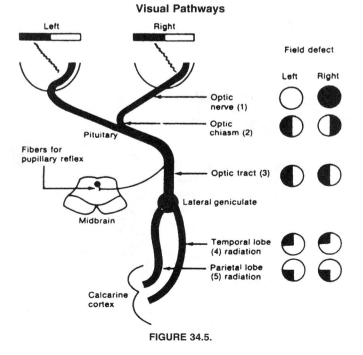

FIGURE 34.5.

atrophy secondary to prolonged increased intracranial pressure. The optic nerve also may be affected by vascular processes such as giant-cell arteritis and amaurosis fugax.

2. *Bitemporal hemianopsia* is found classically in the pituitary tumors secondary to pressure on the optic chiasm. Nonhomonymous field defects usually imply lesions near the chiasm. Remember, concentric tunnel vision may be seen in hysterical blindness.

3. *Homonymous hemianopsia* implies a lesion posterior to the chiasm. It may involve optic tract or optic radiations emanating from the lateral geniculate body (or the lateral geniculate itself). The closer a lesion is to the lateral geniculate, the smaller it can be and still produce a homonymous hemianopsia. Occlusions of the posterior cerebral artery usually produce homonymous hemianopsia with sparing of the macula.

4. The *optic radiations* fan out from the lateral geniculate and travel in the temporal and parietal lobes before reaching their destination in the occipital lobe. Lesions in the temporal lobe may give a homonymous superior field defect if the optic radiations are affected. Similarly, a lesion in the parietal lobe may show an inferior homonymous field defect.

5. When one realizes the large territory needed for intact visual fields, it becomes apparent why checking visual fields is a mandatory part of every neurologic examination.

6. With *pupillary response* the pupil depends on input from both the parasympathetic nervous system via the third cranial nerves and sympathetic inputs. Lesions of the third nerve cause dilation of the third nerve; lesion of the sympathetics cause constriction. The pupillary light reflex has an afferent supply from the optic nerve, through the lateral geniculate nucleus of the thalamus, to the midbrain pretectal area to the third nerve. Horner's syndrome is caused by sympathetic disorder of the fibers leading to the pupil and face. Miosis (small pupil), ptosis (partial), and anhidrosis (caused by sweat gland innervation to the face on the same side) are seen in combination. The sympathetics travel from the hypothalamus through the brainstem, spinal cord to Tl or 2, out the roots to near the apex of the lung, up the carotid sheath, and in with the ophthalmic artery.

CRANIAL NERVES

Remember, the first and second cranial nerves lie outside the brainstem. The third and fourth are in the midbrain, fifth through eighth are in the pons, and ninth through twelfth are in the medulla (Fig. 34.6).

I—olfactory, in mesial cortex; rhinencephalon. Smell.

II—optic nerve, enters at lateral geniculate body. Visual function.

III—oculomotor nerve; midbrain. Innervates medial, superior, and inferior rectus; inferior oblique; lid elevator; and pupil.

CRANIAL NERVES

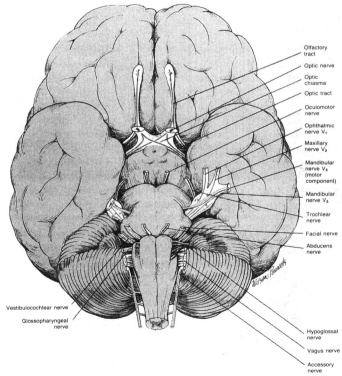

FIGURE 34.6. Cranial nerves. (Reproduced with permission of Ms. Linda Wilson-Pauwels and B. C. Decker, Inc., Hamilton, Ontario, Canada.)

IV—trochlear nerve; midbrain. Innervates superior oblique, brings eye down and in.

V—trigeminal; pons (and medulla). Supplies muscles of mastication, facial sensation, corneal reflex.

VI—abducens; pons. Supplies lateral rectus, brings eye outward.

VII— facial. Supplies facial movements, tearing, and salivation.

VIII—auditory. Supplies hearing and vestibular function.

IX—glossopharyngeal. Supplies palatal sensation.

X—vagus. Supplies muscles of swallowing, autonomic parasympathetics to internal organs.

XI—spinal accessory nerve. Supplies sternocleidomastoid and trapezius muscles.

XII—hypoglossal. Supplies muscles of the tongue.

Midbrain

The most prominent disturbance in the midbrain (cranial nerves III to IV) generally involves the third nerve nucleus or exiting fibers, producing a dilated pupil and ophthalmoplegia (Fig. 34.7). Lesions affecting the area of the midbrain just below the superior colliculus produce difficulty with upward gaze, convergence, and pupillary light reflexes (Parinaud's syndrome). A tumor pressing on the superior colliculus may present in this way (e.g., pinealoma).

Lesions of the red nucleus produce contralateral ataxia and tremor (rubral tremor). The substantia nigra is located at this level and plays an important role in Parkinson's disease.

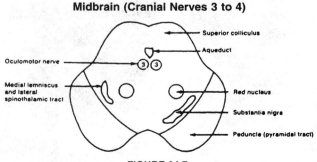

Midbrain (Cranial Nerves 3 to 4)

FIGURE 34.7.

The fourth nerve nucleus also is located in the midbrain at a lower level and seldom is involved alone. When it is involved alone (e.g., because of trauma), fourth nerve injury causes a head tilt.

Fibers from the optic tract are concerned with the pupillary response synapse in the region of the third nerve nucleus. Lesions in the midbrain may impair pupillary reaction to direct light but leave contraction to accommodation intact.

Pons

The fibers of the seventh (facial) nerve sweep around the sixth nerve (lateral rectus) before exiting from the pons (cranial nerves V to VIII) (Fig. 34.8). Thus, a lesion at this level often produces a VI and VII nerve paralysis on the same side.

In the basic structure of the pons, medial involvement produces motor dysfunction and internuclear ophthalmoplegia or gaze palsy to the side of the lesion. Lateral involvement causes pain and temperature dysfunction.

Vertical nystagmus is a sign of brainstem dysfunction at the level of the pontomedullary junction or upper midbrain (unless the patient is taking barbiturates). Eighth nerve nuclei include cochlear and vestibular components.

The *trigeminal nerve* exits from the middle of the pons and if involved at this level produces face pain and ipsilateral loss of the corneal reflex. In high pontine lesions, pain and sensory loss are contralateral to the lesion in the face and extremities. Below the

Pons (Cranial nerves 5 to 8)

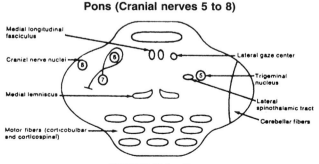

FIGURE 34.8. Pons.

high pons, pain and temperature senses are lost ipsilaterally in the face and contralaterally in the limbs.

Lesions of the *medical longitudinal fasciculus* (MLF) result in an internuclear ophthalmoplegia. If the right MLF is involved, there is difficulty with right eye adduction, as well as nystagmus in the abducting left eye when the patient looks to the left.

Medulla

The most commonly encountered vascular syndrome affecting the medulla (cranial nerves IX to XII) is the *lateral medullary* (*Wallenberg syndrome*) (see Chapter 16), which defines a major portion of the dysfunction that can be seen with medullary involvement (Fig. 34.9). (Medial structures are unaffected: pyramids, medial lemniscus, and twelfth nerve nucleus.)

Remember that the *seventh (facial) nerve is not in the medulla*. Thus, if facial weakness is present, there must be dysfunction at the level of the pons or above.

When *descending sympathetic fibers* are involved, an ipsilateral Horner's syndrome (ptosis, small pupil, and facial anhidrosis) results.

Cranial nerve nuclei include the following:

Twelfth (hypoglossal): Unilateral involvement of nucleus causes fasciculations on that side; when the tongue is protruded, it deviates to the side of the lesion.

Medulla (Cranial Nerves 9 to 12)

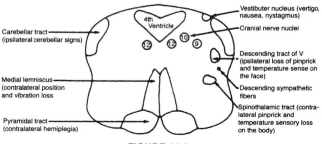

FIGURE 34.9.

Tenth (vagus) and ninth (glossopharyngeal): These innervate the laryngeal and pharyngeal musculature; dysphagia is prominent when they are involved.

SPINAL CORD

Vascular Supply

The *anterior spinal artery* (5) supplies the entire cord except for the dorsal columns. Thus, the anterior spinal artery syndrome produces paralysis and loss of pain and temperature sense; position and vibratory sense are preserved (Fig. 34.10).

The clinical correlation follows:

- Subacute combined system disease affects 1 and 3.
- Amyotrophic lateral sclerosis affects 3 and 4.
- Tabes dorsalis affects 1.
- Multiple sclerosis affects 1, 2, and 3 (alone or in combination).
- Poliomyelitis affects 4.
- Brown-Séquard syndrome (hemisection of cord) produces ipsilateral paralysis, ipsilateral loss of vibration and position

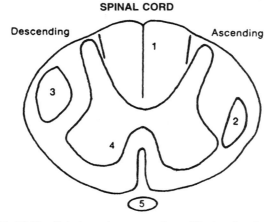

FIGURE 34.10. Spinal cord cross-section: *(1)* dorsal columns; *(2)* spinothalamic tracts; *(3)* corticospinal tracts; *(4)* anterior horns; *(5)* anterior spinal artery.

sense, and contralateral loss of sensation to pinprick and temperature.

Dorsal columns (1) carry position and vibratory sense; fibers rise ipsilaterally and cross in the medulla. These columns are laminated, but the lamination is usually of little clinical importance.

Lateral spinothalamic tract (2) carries pain and temperature sensation. These fibers cross on entering the cord; a cord lesion affecting them produces a contralateral loss. They are laminated with sacral fibers most laterally placed. Thus, an expanding process in the center of the cord gives sacral sparing (pinprick and temperature sensory loss are least prominent in the sacral area).

Descending Tracts

Lateral corticospinal tract (3) carries motor fibers that synapse at the anterior horn cells. The fibers have crossed in the medulla already. A lesion or pressure on the corticospinal tract causes weakness, spasticity, hyperreflexia, and up-going toes.

Anterior horn cells (4) are lower motor neurons. A lesion here produces weakness, muscle wasting, fasciculations, and loss of reflexes and tone (Fig. 34.11).

Suggested Reading

Adams RD, Victor M, Ropper AH. *Principles of neurology*, 6th ed. New York: McGraw-Hill, 1997.

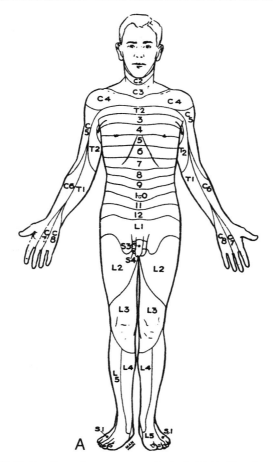

FIGURE 34.11. Dermatome sensory chart. **A.** Right. The dermatomes from the anterior view.

(continued on next page)

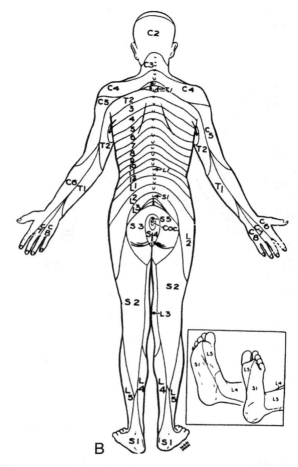

FIGURE 34.11 *(Continued)* **B.** Left. Dermatomes from the posterior view. (From Keegan JJ, Garrett FD. The segmental distribution of the cutaneous nerves in the limbs of man. *Anat Rec* 1948;102:409. Reprinted with permission of the Wistar Institute Press, Philadelphia.)

TABLE 34.1. Crossings in the Nervous System[a]

Pathway	Function	Crosses	Interpretation
Pyramidal tract	Motor	Lower medulla	Lesion below crossing gives ipsilateral signs
Spinothalamic tract	Pain and temperature (body)	On entry to spinal cord	Lesion is always contralateral to pain and temperature loss (except in face)
Spinal tract of fifth (V) nerve	Pain and temperature (face)	Midpons (runs throughout medulla)	If lesion is in medulla or lower pons—ipsilateral loss; above midpons—contralateral loss
Spinal dorsal columns	Position and vibration	Lower medulla	Lesion below crossing gives ipsilateral signs
Cerebellar tracts	Coordination of movement	Crosses twice (on entry to cerebellum and in midbrain)	Because of the "double crossing" lesion of cerebellum or cerebellar tracts, usually produce signs and symptoms ipsilateral to lesion
Gaze fibers	Coordinates lateral gaze	Midpons	See Figure 34.2 for interpretation
Cranial nerve fibers	Cranial nerves	Just above cranial nerve	Lesion is ipsilateral when cranial nerve nuclei are involved

[a]Almost all major pathways in the nervous system cross. Much of the understanding of neuroanatomy relates to knowing where these tracts cross and, thus, at which level the nervous system is involved.

Chapter 35

Differential Diagnoses in Neurology

Although long lists of differential diagnoses are usually unhelpful in clinical neurology, certain signs and symptoms suggest a list of diagnoses. This chapter includes selected topics that are not specifically mentioned in the text but have been found to be particularly useful. The list is not meant to be exhaustive, but it may be helpful to the house officer and encourage him or her to develop and review similar lists for easy reference in other areas of neurology and medicine.

AMNESIA, ACUTE

1. Head injury
2. Postictal amnesia
3. Transient global amnesia
4. Encephalitis
5. Intoxications (e.g., alcohol)
6. Basilar migraine
7. Wernicke's encephalopathy
8. Psychiatric

BRACHIAL PLEXUS LESIONS

1. Idiopathic brachial plexitis
2. Tumor infiltration, especially breast cancer
3. Trauma
4. Radiation plexopathy
5. Postinjection

6. Polyarteritis nodosa, lupus
7. Lyme disease

CRANIAL NERVE PALSIES

1. Cavernous sinus lesion (may involve II, III, IV, V_{1-2}, VI)
2. Base-of-skull disorders
3. Meningeal disorders
4. Idiopathic cranial neuropathy
5. Intrinsic brainstem lesions
6. Vasculitis
7. Carotid dissection
8. Myasthenia gravis

CHOREOATHETOSIS

1. Huntington's disease
2. Sydenham's chorea
3. Birth control pills
4. Pregnancy associated (chorea gravidarum)
5. Stroke—basal ganglia
6. Lupus
7. Cerebral palsy
8. Carbon monoxide
9. Sinemet, other dopamine agonists
10. Wilson's disease

FASCICULATIONS

1. Motor neuron disease
2. Chronic root compression
3. Benign fasciculation syndrome, especially in athletes and health care workers
4. Polio
5. Syringomyelia
6. Metabolic disorders (thyrotoxicosis)

HORNER'S SYNDROME

1. Brainstem lesion
2. Lower trunk brachial plexus lesion (apex of lung mass)

3. Cord lesion
4. Neck lesion
5. Carotid lesion
6. Hypothalamic lesion

MYELOPATHY

Acute

1. Epidural metastases
2. Ischemic, embolic
3. Trauma
4. Lupus, vasculitis
5. Toxins (arsenic)
6. Multiple sclerosis (MS)
7. Arteriovenous malformation—with bleed
8. Transverse myelitis

Chronic

1. MS
2. Slow-growing tumors
3. Primary lateral sclerosis
4. Deficiencies (e.g., vitamin B_{12})
5. Spinal stenosis

MYOCLONUS

1. Anoxia
2. Uremia
3. Meningitis
4. Encephalitis
5. Cephalosporins and penicillins in patients with renal failure

RECURRENT MENINGITIS

1. Mollaret's meningitis
2. Bacterial with compromised barriers (cerebrospinal fluid leak, dural sinus)
3. Parameningeal focus
4. Drug induced (nonsteroidal medication)

5. Chemical
6. Chemotherapy

NEUROPATHY WITH "BURNING FEET"

1. Diabetes
2. Toxins including drugs
3. Human immunodeficiency virus associated

PTOSIS

1. Sympathetic lesion
2. Migraine
3. Cluster headache
4. Myopathy
5. Congenital ptosis
6. Third nerve lesion

RADICULOPATHY—ACUTE

1. Disc herniation
2. Herpes zoster
3. Diabetes
4. Tumor infiltration

"WASTED HANDS"

1. Motor neuron disorders
2. Plexus lesions (lower trunk)
3. C8–T1 root lesion
4. Cervical root compression
5. Compression neuropathies (e.g., carpal tunnel)
6. Syringomyelia or other cord lesion affecting lower motor neuron
7. Distal myopathies

Subject Index

Page numbers in *italics* denote figures; page numbers followed by a t denote tables.